COMMON SYMPTOMS OF DISEASE

WT 100
HOP

N2160

This book is due for return on or before the last date shown below.

31. JUL 1981

-7. SEP. 1990

19 JUN 91

23. APR. 1982

-8. JUL. 1982

09 April 83

NOV. 1984

20. OCT. 1989

Common Symptoms of Disease in the Elderly

H. M. HODKINSON
MA DM FRCP

*Professor of Geriatric Medicine
Royal Postgraduate Medical School,
Hammersmith Hospital, London*

SECOND EDITION

BLACKWELL SCIENTIFIC PUBLICATIONS
OXFORD LONDON EDINBURGH MELBOURNE

© 1976, 1980 by
Blackwell Scientific Publications
Editorial offices:
Osney Mead, Oxford OX2 0EL
8 John Street, London WC1N 2ES
9 Forrest Road, Edinburgh EH1 2QH
214 Berkeley Street, Carlton
   Victoria 3053, Australia

All rights reserved. No part of this
publication may be reproduced,
stored in a retrieval system, or
transmitted, in any form or by any
means, electronic, mechanical,
photocopying, recording or otherwise
without the prior permission of
the copyright owner

First published 1976
Second edition 1980

Printed and bound in Great Britain by
Billing and Sons Limited
Guildford, London and Worcester

DISTRIBUTORS

USA
   Blackwell Mosby Book Distributors
   11830 Westline Industrial Drive
   St Louis, Missouri 63141

Canada
   Blackwell Mosby Book Distributors
   86 Northline Road, Toronto
   Ontario M4B 3E5

Australia
   Blackwell Scientific Book
   Distributors
   214 Berkeley Street, Carlton
   Victoria 3053

British Library Cataloguing
in Publication Data

Hodkinson, Henry Malcolm
   Common symptoms of disease in
   the elderly—2nd ed.
   1. Geriatrics   2. Semiology
   I. Title
   618.9'7'072 RC953

ISBN 0-632-00622-6

CONTENTS

	Preface	vii
1	How disease differs in old age	1
2	Non-specific presentations of illness	6
3	Presentations with mental symptoms	21
4	Rheumatic and locomotor symptoms	35
5	Falls, faints and turns	47
6	Cardio-respiratory presentations	58
7	Alimentary symptoms	71
8	Urinary symptoms	88
9	Neurological symptoms	95
10	The special senses	106
11	The skin	114
12	Symptoms due to drugs	120
	References	133
	Index	137

PREFACE TO FIRST EDITION

Professor Illingworth's popular book *Common Symptoms of Disease in Children* has firmly demonstrated the value of a book written from the standpoint of symptomatology. More recently Dr Fowler's illuminating book *Common Symptoms of Disease in Adults* has followed. It seems worthwhile to extend this approach to the elderly, whose symptomatology may be markedly different from that of earlier adult life so that the non-specialist may find himself in considerable diagnostic difficulties.

The present work seeks to emphasise those areas where there are particularly marked or important alterations of symptomatology in the elderly patient. Comprehensiveness has been subordinated to this aim, so that the book may be regarded as complementary to *Common Symptoms of Disease in Adults*.

The alteration of symptoms in old age partly reflects the confusing effects of multiple disease but the alteration of responses to physical illness is frequent so that, for example, fever, pain or leucocytosis may be unexpectedly absent whilst mental symptoms may often be the main manifestation of physical disease. Insidious presentations are particularly common and this, coupled with the general tendency of the elderly to be stoically uncomplaining and to over-readily attribute their symptoms to mere old age, means that the doctor dealing with elderly patients has to be on his mettle if he is not to overlook the diagnosis of treatable disease. I need make no apology for my intentional emphasis on the diagnosis and symptoms of potentially treatable conditions.

The book aims to be a practical one and it is hoped that the reader will be able to read through it in continuity but will equally find it a useful book of reference when confronted with an individual diagnostic problem.

References are deliberately few and preference has been given to readily available sources of useful further reading. I have been somewhat liberal in my interpretation of the word 'symptom' in that I have considered readily observed changes in general appearance, behaviour or mobility such as are apparent before the patient is formally examined even though they may not be complained of as symptoms by the patient.

London, 1976   *Malcolm Hodkinson*

PREFACE TO SECOND EDITION

The favourable reception of the first edition has encouraged me to make no major changes in preparing a second edition. I have tried to keep to the same general pattern and to resist the temptation to enlarge the book to any degree.

I have contented myself with necessary revision and in providing more up to date references. I have corrected some minor inaccuracies which were pointed out by helpful colleagues.

London, 1979   *Malcolm Hodkinson*

1

HOW DISEASE DIFFERS IN OLD AGE

Children are not simply miniature adults, and paediatric medicine shows many important differences from adult medicine. At the other extreme of life, the elderly similarly show many modifications of patterns of disease as compared with younger adult patients. These differences characteristic of geriatric medicine combine with the difficulties of history taking and physical examination in the elderly and render accurate diagnosis more difficult. Accurate diagnosis is no less essential in the elderly than in any other age group however, for there is much treatable disease to be found and much else can be helped if not cured.

Multiple disease

Perhaps the most striking differences between the younger adult and the elderly patient is the finding that whereas the younger patient has but a single diagnosis, multiple diagnoses are usual in the old. This difference calls for a major reorientation of diagnostic thinking as traditional medical teaching, reflecting the medicine of younger adults, has laid great stress on the importance of bringing together all the findings of history, examination and investigation within the embrace of a single unifying diagnosis. Such an approach is quite inappropriate to the elderly patient and will grossly mislead the clinician.

Old people bear the permanent defects due to past injuries,

illnesses and operations. They accumulate diseases that can be controlled but not cured such as pernicious anaemia or myxoedema, diseases that disable but do not kill such as osteoarthritis, osteoporosis or cataract and other potentially lethal but chronic diseases such as atherosclerosis, diverticulosis or diabetes. Many diseases have a frequency which rises with age: malignancies, stroke, depression, Parkinson's disease, senile dementia and fracture of the femur are a few important examples. New diseases arise against a background of pre-existing diseases and disabilities but also of a slow decline in the functional capacity of most body systems resulting from physiological or non-pathological age changes. Thus respiratory reserve, renal function and many homoeostatic mechanisms such as temperature regulation and the control of blood pressure, posture and osmolality all show steady if undramatic declines with age.

Multiple factors may combine to produce modified clinical presentations. Furthermore, multiple diseases and disabilities may summate and interact so that a number of minor lesions which would be of little consequence individually may together be important. Thus heart failure may often be due to the combined effects of several 'trivial' pathologies as Pomerance (1972) has shown. For similar reasons, complications of the primary illness are far more likely in the aged. Important examples are the frequent development of thromboembolism, dehydration, pressure sores, hypostatic pneumonia, immobility and contractures in the elderly and the greatly increased hazards of drug therapy.

Altered responses to illness

Body responses to illness may be considerably modified in the elderly. Altered pain and temperature responses are particularly noteworthy and are discussed below. The reticuloendothelial system is less responsive so that leucocytosis is less often encountered or when present is less in extent. Lymphangitis and lymphadenopathy seldom develop in infections. Mental confusion, an increased pulse rate or other unobtrusive manifestations may instead be the main indications of infection.

Pain

The elderly complain of pain less often than might be expected. Conditions which are usually accompanied by severe pain in the young may be totally painless in old age. Thus painless myocardial infarction is far more common than is the 'typical' presentation with crushing chest pain and shock. Similarly many osteoporotic old people have collapsed vertebrae but have no corresponding history of back pain.

The relative infrequency of the complaint of pain in the elderly can be attributed in part to their greater stoicism, and pain may be more readily forgotten where there is mental impairment. The main difference would seem to lie in some change in the physiology of pain appreciation in old age. Even when pain is experienced, elderly patients often find themselves unable to describe it accurately. Such description as is offered seldom conforms to the textbook description so that, for example, angina is often grossly atypical.

Some old patients are exceptions to the general rule however, and complain long and loud of pains all over the body. Such multiple complaints of pain should suggest strongly the possibility of hypochondriacal symptoms in a depressed patient.

Changes in the severity or character of chronic pain should also excite special interest. It is all too easy to disregard such changes and so overlook, for example, the development of fractured femur in a severely arthritic patient.

Temperature

Experimental studies show that thermoregulation tends to deteriorate with age (Collins *et al.* 1977). This can be seen clinically both in the way the elderly are less likely to respond to illness by elevation of temperature and in the increased tendency to develop hypothermia.

The failure to develop a raised temperature in response to illness, particularly infection, is a very common one in the old. Even when temperature is affected, the rise tends to be less dramatic and rigors are very uncommon. Chest infections frequently fail to give rise to any temperature elevation and the clinician must rely on more subtle signs and symptoms such as a modest increase in pulse rate or slight tachypnoea and be aware that the onset of mental confusion is frequently due to this cause. Even when grave infections are present, for example empyema, pyarthrosis, subphrenic abscess or peritonitis, temperature may not rise and the presentation may be insidious or non-specific. As there may not be a leucocyte response either, diagnosis is often very difficult. A high index of suspicion is needed and, for example, it is advisable to carry out a diagnostic aspiration of pleural effusions when the patient seems more ill than would be expected but is afebrile, if the possibility of empyema is not to be overlooked. Blood cultures are often of value in such situations, for severe infections may be accompanied by bacteraemia although there is no fever, whilst subacute bacterial endocarditis and septicaemias are far from rare (Denham & Goodwin 1977).

'Missing' diseases

Whilst almost all diseases may occur in old age, some diseases are surprisingly uncommon. Some of these represent lethal diseases which develop in middle life so that susceptible individuals fail to reach the older age groups. Thus severe hypertension and severe bronchitis and emphysema, though common in middle life, are rarely seen in old age though mild forms are not infrequent.

Infections also have a different pattern of incidence. Thus many viral diseases are seldom seen, presumably due to the prolonged retention of acquired immunity; infective hepatitis is rare for example. A high degree of susceptibility remains where this is not so as in the case of new strains of influenza which may produce devastating epidemics in elderly patient populations. Herpes zoster is particularly common in the elderly.

Some reactions to infection are rarely seen such as acute glomerulonephritis or erythema nodosum. Such changes presumably reflect alterations in the immune status of the elderly.

It is difficult to explain why some locomotor conditions such as prolapsed intervertebral disc, frozen shoulder or brachalgia due to cervical spondylosis, which are very common in late middle life and which have a degenerative basis, should be so uncommon in old age.

Conclusion

The presentation of illness in old age is often misleadingly different from that in earlier age groups. Disease is often multiple, multiple minor pathologies may combine to result in major problems, disease incidences alter with age and response to illness is dramatically altered in later life. Instead of familiar indicators of illness such as pain and fever, greater emphasis must be placed on less obvious signs and symptoms such as slight shortness of breath, a somewhat fast respiratory rate or a quickened pulse. Many illnesses present in an entirely non-specific way or with mental changes, and the next two chapters will deal with these important patterns of disease in old age.

In addition, diagnosis in old age is complicated by the increased difficulties of obtaining a satisfactory history and of physical examination. Furthermore, the elderly are prone to minimise their symptoms; they too readily accept them as being their expected lot. They are particularly likely to fail to seek medical attention promptly or at all (Williamson *et al.* 1964).

2
NON-SPECIFIC PRESENTATIONS OF ILLNESS

Illness in old age often presents as an insidious and progressive deterioration. This may comprise declining social competence, appetite, initiative and drive, together with growing frailty, loss of weight and an increased likelihood of falls. There is often some overlap with the psychiatric presentations considered in the following chapter in that apathy, deteriorating memory and mental confusion may also be present.

To facilitate discussion of these non-specific presentations it is convenient to consider the diagnostic possibilities under a number of very general headings, 'senility', 'slowing up', 'going off his feet', anorexia, weight loss, fatigue and general weakness and 'feeling the cold'. It will be appreciated that there is considerable overlap between these very loose categories and that many could be equally well covered by the term 'failure to thrive' which can usefully be borrowed from paediatrics.

'SENILITY'

To the geriatrician, use of the term 'senility' is rather like a red rag to a bull! This is because it has been used as an alternative to proper diagnosis in the past. It has tended to be indicative of the mistaken attitude that accurate diagnosis was superfluous in an old person as nothing useful could be achieved by treatment.

Senility is not a diagnosis then; rather it should be a diagnostic challenge to find the real cause of an insidious, non-specific deterioration in the physical or physical and mental health of an old person. So if we accept the use of 'senility' in this more constructive sense, what are the more important diagnostic possibilities?

The dementing processes, notably senile dementia and arteriosclerotic dementia, are important possibilities but are liable to be seriously overdiagnosed. The serious pitfall of overlooking a somatic cause for the old person's deterioration by too readily adopting these diagnoses must be avoided. The natural history of the illness is particularly relevant. Senile dementia has a long history of many years of slow and steady mental deterioration, physical deterioration being usual only in the advanced stages of the disease when dementia is profound. Arteriosclerotic dementia, perhaps better termed multi-infarct dementia, also tends to run a lengthy course with step-wise deterioration due to a series of cerebral infarctions which may or may not be clinically recognisable at the time. In contrast, deterioration due to somatic disease is likely to have a much shorter time course and the patient to be more obviously ill or frail.

Depression is another important and treatable possible cause of non-specific decline. The cardinal symptoms of anorexia and early waking should always be the subject of inquiry. A depressed appearance often draws attention to the diagnosis and it is important not to be misled by hypochondriacal symptoms suggesting physical disease. Depression and physical illness may not infrequently coexist as the latter may trigger the development of the depressive illness.

Malignant disease often presents non-specifically, the commoner primary sites being lung, breast, prostate, colon, rectum and stomach. Carcinoma of the pancreas, though less common, is particularly likely to present insidiously. Prompt diagnosis of malignant disease is important for some neoplasms are amenable to surgery, particularly carcinoma of the colon, whilst hormonal therapy may have much to offer even in advanced cases of cancer of breast or prostate.

Endocrine causes should be considered. Myxoedema is quite common in the elderly and may often not be recognised clinically. Bahemuka and Hodkinson (1975) found that 2·2% of elderly patients had unsuspected hypothyroidism when routine laboratory tests were carried out. The patients discovered in this way did not show the textbook picture of myxoedema but had presented with apathy, depression, mental and physical slowing and a variety of other non-specific complaints which improved after commencement of treatment. Similarly they found the prevalence of hyperthyroidism to be over 1% and here again the presentation was usually atypical and unobtrusive, in some corresponding to what has been described as 'apathetic' thyrotoxicosis (*Lancet* 1970). Again the condition is eminently treatable. Diabetes is very common in old age. Denham (1972) found over 5% of geriatric patients to have diabetes which had been previously unknown, a further 8% having previously diagnosed diabetes. Few present with typical symptoms of weight loss, thirst and polyuria. Non-specific presentations are common in contrast and may precede the development of ketosis or of non-ketotic hypersomolar coma. Denham showed that random blood sugar was a far better screening test for the recognition of diabetes than was urinalysis as quite a proportion of the diabetics showed no glycosuria because of a raised renal threshold for glucose.

Uraemia and anaemia are other important causes of 'failure to thrive' and again are most reliably recognised by laboratory screening tests. It can thus be appreciated that laboratory profile screening of elderly patients showing a non-specific deterioration in their health is of great potential value and should preferably include thyroid screening tests such as T4 and T3-uptake determinations.

Central nervous system disease may also present insidiously. Parkinsonism is common in old age but, as tremor is often absent or inconspicuous, may be overlooked if the characteristic facies is not noticed and if rigidity is not sought for. As L-dopa therapy can give such gratifying improvements, the diagnosis is an important one which should be actively sought. Observation of gait may often be a useful clue. The head-drop test as a test for neck rigidity (Wartenberg 1952) can be useful, especially when limb tone is difficult to assess because of poor cooperation. The patient lies on his back without a pillow with the examiner's hand under the head. When the patient has relaxed, the examiner suddenly tosses up the head. In the normal subject the head falls back rapidly but rigidity slows the fall markedly. The glabella tap sign, on the other hand, is not of much value as it is often positive in elderly subjects without parkinsonism.

Slowly developing peripheral neuropathy should be considered and, if sensory symptoms are inconspicuous, may easily be overlooked. Loss of touch sensation is important as absent ankle and, less often, knee jerks and diminution of vibration sense may sometimes be found in apparently normal old people so adding to the difficulties of the interpretation of the C.N.S. signs (Prakash & Stern 1973). Diabetes and carcinoma of the bronchus are perhaps the commonest causes of peripheral neuropathy in old age but subacute combined degeneration of the cord with peripheral neuropathy due to vitamin B_{12} deficiency should be remembered as a less common but easily treatable alternative possibility.

Chronic infections are yet another cause of a non-specific decline. Subacute bacterial endocarditis should be thought of when the patient has a cardiac murmur and any possibility of the diagnosis should lead to the taking of blood cultures as prognosis is good if the disease is recognised and treated but is otherwise extremely grave. Tuberculosis must not be forgotten; indeed it is more likely to be missed in old age than in any other age group. Miliary tuberculosis, particularly, may have a misleadingly vague clinical picture.

Finally, iatrogenic causes of illness must be borne in mind. Drug side effects will be fully considered in Chapter 12, but here it is relevant to mention such examples as oversedation due to the injudicious use of tranquillisers or hypnotics, depression due to reserpine or methyl-dopa or hyponatraemia or hypoglycaemia associated with the use of chlorpropamide.

'SLOWING UP' AND 'GOING OFF HIS FEET'

Here again, as with 'senility', we are concerned with a non-specific mode of presentation but with a greater emphasis on loss of mobility. Many of the diagnostic possibilities considered above are again relevant here therefore.

When an elderly patient presents with deteriorating mobility it is useful to attempt to roughly classify the difficulty before attempting detailed diagnosis. So we can try to decide whether the deterioration is due to general debility and frailty, to poor exercise tolerance, to stiffness, to specific weakness, to pain or to loss of confidence or motivation. A careful history is essential and it is important that one sees the patient walk or attempt to do so.

General debility and frailty

Here we again need to consider the diseases discussed under 'senility'. In addition we should pay special regard to a number of conditions which may produce generalised muscle weakness. Osteomalacia may be accompanied by a proximal muscle weakness; indeed this may be a striking feature of the illness on occasions, and may give a typical waddling gait and to particular difficulty in rising from a chair. It should be strongly considered in old women who have had partial gastrectomy in the past as this strongly predisposes to osteomalacia. Thyrotoxicosis may also be accompanied by myopathy which is similarly reversible by treatment. Myopathy may occasionally occur in malignant disease. Weakness may be a prominent feature in hyponatraemia which may be due to therapy with chlorpropamide or diuretics or to the syndrome of inappropriate secretion of antidiuretic-hormone, SIADH (Bartter & Schwartz 1967), which may complicate a variety of clinical conditions such as chest infection, trauma, cerebral tumours but is also sometimes found in myxoedema. Hypokalaemia is thought to be common in the elderly (Judge & MacLeod 1968); dietary lack plays a potentially important role but it may also be due to diuretic therapy or to abnormal losses from the gut as in diarrhoea or carcinoma of the rectum or to renal loss in diabetic pre-coma, and may also result in gross weakness.

Poor exercise tolerance

Obesity, heart failure, emphysema, pulmonary fibrosis or anaemia may all limit mobility because of shortness of breath which the patient has not complained of specifically. Silent myocardial infarction and small pulmonary emboli may also be responsible.

Stiffness

The important possibility of parkinsonism has already been referred to. It leads to stiffness, slow movements and often to a liability to fall. Difficulty in moving in bed or of rising from a chair may be more striking than the degree of difficulty in walking. Parkinsonism is usually idiopathic but the possibility of it being drug induced should not be forgotten. Phenothiazine tranquillisers all have this potential side effect, longer acting members of the group are particularly troublesome; prochlorperazine (Stemetil), often given for a minor complaint of giddiness, is a noteworthy offender!

Stiffness may be due to spasticity as in pseudobulbar palsy due to bilateral minor strokes which may have developed unobtrusively or to motor neurone disease which is not rare in old age (Hodkinson 1972). Subacute combined degeneration of the cord is uncommon but is important because of its treatable nature. Paraparesis or quadriparesis due to a variety of cord lesions are occasionally seen. Provided that the nervous system is properly examined as a routine, none of these C.N.S. conditions should be overlooked.

Alternatively, stiffness may be due to skeletal disease. Osteoarthritis is very common in old age, indeed some degree of osteoarthritis is virtually ubiquitous and it is rare indeed for overweight old women not to have quite severe osteoarthritis of the knees. Osteoarthritis of the hips is less common than involvement of the knees but tends to result in far more stiffness and disability. The characteristic gait and the special difficulty of rising from a chair, particularly when it is of low seat height, may draw attention to the diagnosis when there is no complaint of pain. Rheumatoid arthritis is less frequent than osteoarthritis but still quite common, particular in elderly women. It is usually clinically 'burnt out' rather than active and accompanied by much secondary osteoarthritic change. Occasionally rheumatoid arthritis may commence in old age and may be accompanied by considerable malaise and weight loss. Psoriatic arthropathy, ankylosing spondylitis or Reiter's syndrome may also sometimes be seen but usually represent disease which originated in earlier life.

The possibility of a femoral fracture being overlooked in the arthritic patient has already been alluded to. This is most likely in an old case of rheumatoid arthritis where severe osteoporosis is a common feature, especially if steroid therapy has been given, so that fracture may result from relatively minor trauma.

Specific weakness

Minor weakness from a stroke which has occurred unnoticed or from a peripheral neuropathy may be the final event which takes away mobility in a frail patient. Such occurrences should present little diagnostic difficulty.

Pain

Pain, though not specifically complained of by the patient, may be responsible for deterioration in mobility. Thus angina of effort, which may be more a feeling of discomfort or of oppression rather than a typical pain, or intermittent claudication may curtail walking. Painful or uncomfortable feet may also prevent mobility. Thus large onychogryphoses may describe almost a full circle so that they come to press on the sole of the foot. Neglected corns or calluses or painful bunions may similarly discourage ambulation.

Arthritis has already been considered as a cause of stiffness, but equally may interfere with mobility because of pain.

Loss of confidence and problems of motivation

Mobility may deteriorate because of loss of confidence and this is particularly likely in old people who are afraid of *falling* or who suffer from *giddiness,* problems that will be discussed more fully in Chapter 5. Demented or depressed patients may become immobile because of their poor motivation. Overprotective attitudes in relatives or doctors may contribute: one has met frail-looking but essentially healthy old ladies who had not walked for years simply because their family and doctor had convinced them that they were not capable of it! Even a short period of rest in bed for some episode of intercurrent illness may be enough to destroy confidence and mobility in some poorly motivated or overanxious old people.

ANOREXIA

Anorexia must be distinguished from other causes of a failure to take adequate food such as dysphagia, dyspepsia, nausea and severe dyspnoea—all of which are considered more fully later. In addition there are psychiatric reasons for a failure to eat adequately such as severe dementia, self-neglect or the delusional belief that food is poisoned which again do not amount to true anorexia.

When true anorexia is present one must consider, first and foremost, the possibility of depression. This is the diagnosis most often missed in elderly patients but would more often be recognised if due attention were always paid to its cardinal symptoms of anorexia and early waking. Anorexia may also be a feature of anxiety states though these are not often seen in an acute or florid form in old age.

Loss of appetite very often occurs as a temporary phenomenon in acute illness but equally is often seen in any severe and more persistent illness. It is frequently a facet of an otherwise non-specific illness and is very common indeed in the terminal stages of illness.

Alternatively, anorexia may point more specifically to gastro-intestinal disease and is particularly characteristic in carcinoma of the stomach which may otherwise present in a totally non-specific way. Patients who have had a partial gastrectomy in the past may never regain their appetite again. Anorexia may also be a prominent feature in pernicious anaemia, presumably as a manifestation of the atrophic gastritis that is present. Similarly the chronic gastritis of alcoholism may lead to marked loss of appetite. Alcoholism is often denied by elderly patients and may remain unsuspected until relatives, neighbours or social workers reveal the true state of affairs. One way in which the diagnosis may be indicated is the finding of an otherwise unexplained elevation of mean corpuscular volume (M.C.V.) on a routine blood count.

Metabolic disturbances may cause severe loss of appetite. This may be a prominent feature of the otherwise unobtrusive changes in progressive uraemia and may also be seen in hepatic dysfunction.

Finally, drugs may produce anorexia, the main culprit being digitalis.

LOSS OF WEIGHT

Clearly any of the conditions enumerated above which result in a diminished food intake will result in weight loss if present for a sufficient length of time. Moreover, recurrent episodes of acute illness giving temporary anorexia may also lead to a substantial loss of weight.

In a number of illnesses the weight loss seems to be greater than would be expected from the degree of diminution of food intake. This is particularly true of malignant disease, especially of carcinoma of the stomach or pancreas but may also be noted in chronic infections or chronic inflammatory disease such as active rheumatoid arthritis. Chronic and severe cardiac failure may lead to gross weight loss, 'cardiac cachexia', as may the presence of large pressure sores.

There are other instances where weight loss appears despite what appears to be a reasonable food intake. In younger age groups thyrotoxicosis, diabetes or Simmond's disease spring to mind as possible explanations in such circumstances but are rarely in fact responsible in elderly patients. Malabsorption syndromes are, however, seen from time to time. That following partial gastrectomy is perhaps the most common. Coeliac disease is occasionally seen. Other occasional causes are chronic pancreatitis, internal fistulae as complications of diverticulitis or gastrointestinal neoplasm, small intestinal diverticulosis (Clark 1972) and scleroderma.

Sometimes one sees patients with marked involuntary movements who lose weight presumably because of the resulting increase in calorie expenditure. Weight loss is also a feature of the late stages of senile dementia but is difficult to explain.

Sometimes too one sees slow but progressive weight loss in the very old (those over ninety) for which there appears to be no pathological cause. Finally, some patients complain of weight loss which on further enquiry proves to be due to their adherence to some special diet which may have been recommended for dubious reasons.

FATIGUE AND GENERAL WEAKNESS

These symptoms too are commonly a minor facet of an essentially non-specific presentation of illness the many possible causes of which have now been discussed at some length. However, when fatigue and general weakness are more prominent features, some potential causes need to be accorded greater weight. They are more likely as features in chronic infections, in chronic inflammatory diseases, in malignant disease and in anaemias.

In particular one should think of possible endocrine and metabolic causes. Endocrine causes include thyrotoxicosis, hypothyroidism and uncontrolled diabetes. Addison's diasease may also give striking fatigue and weakness but is very uncommon in the elderly. Metabolic causes include uraemia, hyponatraemia and hypokalaemia which have already been considered but also hypercalcaemia. Hypercalcaemia is a far from rare occurrence in elderly patients. The three main causes in order of frequency are firstly carcinoma of the bronchus with secretion of ectopic parathormone-like hormone, secondly cases of carcinomatosis with multiple osteolytic metastases and thirdly true hyperparathyroidism (Grero & Hodkinson 1977).

Myasthenia gravis has fatiguability as its most characteristic feature but is excessively rare in old age.

Finally one should remember the possibility of oversedation with tranquillisers, hypnotics or anti-epileptic drugs as the cause of fatigue and weakness.

FEELING THE COLD

Many frail or ill old people complain of feeling the cold. This probably represents a consequence of their general inactivity with reduction of heat production because of reduced muscular work. Furthermore, insulation may be less efficient if subcutaneous fat is reduced as part of a general loss of weight due to illness.

Feeling the cold is more specifically regarded as a symptom of hypothyroidism but is seldom actually complained of by elderly patients with this disease!

Finally, patients may complain of coldness of the extremities. Coldness of the feet may be due to peripheral vascular disease when absent arterial pulses and dependent cyanosis will be noted. Cold hands may be due to episodes of Raynaud's phenomenon. This is a common manifestation of scleroderma which is not rare in old age. It may be recognised by the acrosclerosis in the fingers, reduced mouth gape and punctate telangectasia around the lips. Rheumatoid arthritis may also be associated with Raynaud's phenomenon.

ROUTINE INVESTIGATION IN THE OLD PERSON WITH NON-SPECIFIC PRESENTATION OF ILLNESS

As illness so often presents non-specifically in old people, the performance of a number of routine screening tests in the sick elderly patient is of great value (Hodkinson 1977). A reasonably thorough battery of tests might usefully include a chest X-ray, a Coulter S blood count, urea and electrolytes, serum albumin and globulin, calcium, phosphate and alkaline phosphatase, a random blood sugar, thyroid function tests (such as T_4 and T_3-uptake) and routine urinalysis.

Chest X-ray

This may reveal many different disease processes but one will be on the lookout particularly for such diagnoses as pneumonias, tuberculosis, pulmonary embolism and primary or secondary neoplasm. Chest X-ray may reveal marked pulmonary oedema even when cardiac failure had not been suspected clinically. Close attention should be paid to the bony structures. Rib fractures are common and may draw attention to the possibility of osteoporosis or osteomalacia. Looser's zones may be seen, most often in the scapula, and confirm the diagnosis of osteomalacia. Bony metastases may reveal the diagnosis of carcinomatosis or myelomatosis.

Blood count

Anaemia is often found in ill old people. Consideration of the very accurate M.C.V. given by the Coulter S count makes initial classification on which further investigation should be based a relatively easy matter. High M.C.V. suggests a macrocytic anaemia which is most likely to be pernicious anaemia but may be due to folate deficiency in a minority of cases. High M.C.V. may also be due to alcohol or may be found in hypoplastic or aplastic anaemia and can be a striking finding in myxoedema (Bahemuka *et al.* 1973). A low M.C.V. indicates iron deficiency anaemia which is usually secondary to blood loss rather than nutritional deficiency. Anaemia with a normal M.C.V. is likely to be associated with renal failure or with chronic infection, neoplasm or inflammatory disease.

Leucocytosis may indicate infection but a high count of abnormal leucocytes may occasionally reveal the diagnosis of leukaemia. Chronic lymphatic leukaemia is the commonest form in old age but acute leukaemias are also seen.

Polycythaemia is occasionally seen and is more often secondary to pulmonary disease than due to polycythaemia rubra vera.

Urea and electrolytes

A high urea may indicate chronic renal failure in which case a low bicarbonate, a high phosphate and perhaps a high potassium are also likely to be found. The urea may be high because of dehydration in which case bicarbonate will usually be normal and haemoglobin high, in contrast to the tendency to develop a normochromic normocytic anaemia in chronic renal failure.

Hyponatraemia and hypokalaemia may be other important findings whose significance has already been discussed.

Albumin and globulin

These can give very useful information. Albumin is a sensitive indicator of constitutional upset and may fall to very low levels in serious illness irrespective of the cause. Some diseases are especially likely to give a low albumin however, for example cirrhosis, rheumatoid arthritis and ulcerative colitis.

A moderate rise in globulin may be seen in a wide range of diseases involving infection or due to malignancy. A more marked elevation of globulin of above 40 g/l should suggest the possibility of myelomatosis and lead to electrophoresis and the search for a monoclonal globulin band and examination of the urine for Bence Jones proteinuria.

Calcium, phosphate and alkaline phosphatase

Here the principal aim is to recognise osteomalacia as this can be most successfully treated. Typically, osteomalacia gives a low calcium and phosphate and an elevated alkaline phosphatase. It is advisable to correct the calcium for protein variation in view of the frequency of disturbances in ill old people. Renal failure may also give rise to hypocalcaemia but leads to elevation of phosphate. If alkaline phosphatase is also raised renal osteomalacia is likely and bone biopsy will be needed to confirm the diagnosis.

Hypercalcaemia may be found and may indicate carcinoma of the bronchus, bony metastases or hyperparathyroidism.

A raised alkaline phosphatase may have many other causes apart from osteomalacia. Important possibilities are liver disease, bony metastases and Paget's disease. Minor elevation of alkaline phosphatase commonly follows fractures and often occurs in rheumatoid arthritis.

Thyroid tests

It is advisable to use two *in vitro* tests together so that a Free-thyroxine-index can be derived as this will eliminate the difficulties due to variations in thyroxine binding proteins. Otherwise interpretation of a single test becomes difficult and misleading because such binding protein changes are very common in ill old people (Jefferys *et al.* 1972). A Free-thyroxine-index calculated from the ratio of T_4 (or P.B.I.) and T_3-uptake is, in contrast, relatively easily interpreted, high values suggesting hyperthyroidism and low ones hypothyroidism. However, abnormal values overlap the normal range so that repeat tests and further confirmatory investigations are usually needed to clinch a diagnosis (Hodkinson 1977).

Random glucose

Denham (1972) has shown that a random mid-morning blood glucose is an efficient screening test for diabetes, those with results above 10·4 mmol/l (185 mg%) having a greater than 50% chance of having diabetes.

Occasionally the random glucose test may show hypoglycaemia. This is most often due to overtreatment with insulin or with oral hypoglycaemic agents in a known diabetic but occasionally a case of spontaneous hypoglycaemia is found.

Urinalysis

Glycosuria is a less effective screen for diabetes than the random blood sugar as false negatives are relatively common in the elderly (Denham 1972). Proteinuria may indicate renal disease such as chronic pyelonephritis or chronic glomerulonephritis. Nephrotic syndrome is very uncommon in old age. Alternatively proteinuria may indicate urinary infection and this possibility should be checked by culture of a mid-stream specimen. Urinary infections are very common, particularly in elderly women.

3
PRESENTATIONS WITH MENTAL SYMPTOMS

FORGETFULNESS

We are all a little forgetful but it is generally accepted that the elderly are somewhat more forgetful. Thus, mild forgetfulness in old age with a tendency to live in the past can be accepted as normal. The danger is that we make too generous an allowance for such changes and overlook pathological memory impairment in an old person. One is particularly likely to fall into this error when the forgetful old person has preserved an excellent social façade. He or she may pass the time of day and engage us in normal polite conversation without arousing any suspicions and yet simple testing of memory may reveal gross disability. This common experience has persuaded many doctors who work with the elderly of the necessity to apply a simple test of orientation and memory as a routine (Denham & Jefferys 1972). One such simple test is shown overleaf (Hodkinson 1972).

Normal old people drop only a mark or two at most on such a test, indeed many will score the maximum. Pathological memory loss is clearly reflected by score loss however.

When abnormal forgetfulness is demonstrable one should not automatically jump to the conclusion that the patient is demented. Senile dementia and arteriosclerotic dementia are, of course important diagnostic possibilities but are only likely where there is a prolonged history of progressive mental deterioration. Some

ABBREVIATED MENTAL TEST SCORE
(Each question scores one mark)

1. Age
2. Time (to nearest hour)
3. Address for recall at end of test—this should be repeated by the patient to ensure it has been heard correctly:
   42 West Street
4. Year
5. Name of hospital
6. Recognition of two persons (doctor, nurse, etc.)
7. Date of birth
8. Year of First World War
9. Name of present Monarch
10. Count backwards 20–1

old people appear to have an exaggerated memory loss which may be very slowly progressive but does not seem to amount to a true dementing process. This has been termed benign senescent forgetfulness (Kral 1962).

One should also be cautious in the interpretation of a low test score when the elderly person, who may have been of relatively low intelligence throughout life, comes from a socially and culturally deprived background. Dementia can only be reliably diagnosed in such individuals if progressive deterioration in mental state can be detected either on the basis of a careful history from friends or relatives or by follow up. Depressed patients may also perform badly on tests of orientation and memory. This sub-group of depressed patients has been termed 'pseudodementia' and should be carefully distinguished from true dementia by the shorter history and the presence of other depressive features such as early waking, anorexia and depressive thoughts or delusions if an important therapeutic opportunity is not to be missed.

When deterioration of memory is recent, it should excite particularly keen diagnostic interest. Milder forms of acute delirium (confusional states) may present with memory impairment as their main feature. Confusional states may be due to a wide range of physical diseases and represent one of the most important differential diagnostic problems of the medicine of old age and offer many opportunities for effective therapeutic intervention. The detailed discussion which follows under the heading of 'confusion' should be referred to.

Memory may deteriorate suddenly after a cerebrovascular accident and, when this involves a 'silent' area of the brain, there may be few or no clinical central nervous system signs to be found. Rapidly deteriorating memory may also be the presenting symptom in a variety of intracranial space-occupying lesions such as glioma, secondary deposit particularly from a bronchial primary, meningioma or subdural haematoma. The latter is an important possibility and offers the chance of effective surgical treatment and must be seriously considered if there is a history of a recent fall with injury to the head, however minor, and if the patient shows fluctuation in the mental state. Skull X-ray may show evidence of midline shift and an isotope brain scan may give more definitive information.

More transient amnesia may follow head injury, grand mal epilepsy or E.C.T. Amnesia is particularly characteristic of Wernicke's encephalopathy due to chronic alcoholism which is occasionally seen in geriatric practice.

Forgetfulness is an important early symptom in hypothyroidism and may point to the diagnosis long before any typical signs or symptoms of myxoedema are to be found. Laboratory screening tests are the only way to recognise hypothyroidism at this stage. If these are not performed routinely they should be freely requested when forgetfulness is part of the clinical presentation and has no obvious explanation.

Finally, forgetfulness may be the main feature of 'hangover' or oversedation due to the injudicious use of tranquillisers, hypnotics, anti-epileptics or other sedative drugs.

CONFUSION

Acute confusion

Acute mental confusion as a presenting symptom holds a central place in the medicine of old age. Its importance cannot be overemphasised for acute confusion is a far more common herald of the onset of physical illness in an old person than are, for example, fever, pain or tachycardia.

Acute confusional states may develop in old people who were previously mentally normal but a large multi-centre study has clearly shown that pre-existing dementia greatly favours their development (Hodkinson 1973). The pattern of a fully developed confusional state is that described by the psychiatric term of acute delirium. This comprises clouding of consciousness, impaired memory, disorientation, restlessness and rambling speech. Sensory stimuli may be misinterpreted and hallucinations, delusions and noisy or aggressive behaviour may occur. There may be undue wakefulness or reversal of diurnal sleep pattern or episodes of drowsiness or coma may supervene. The great majority of the confusional states seen in old people represent very much incomplete versions of this picture of acute delirium.

When a clearly ill old person becomes acutely confused, recognition that this is an acute confusional state is generally obvious. It is when only the mental symptoms are obvious that the underlying physical basis of the disturbance may not be appreciated. This represents a serious error for if the physical disease is recognised and effectively treated, full mental recovery can be anticipated.

An enormous variety of physical illnesses may give rise to confusional states. Particularly potent causes are infections, especially pneumonias and urinary infections, congestive heart failure and left ventricular failure and carcinomatosis (Hodkinson 1973). Acute cerebrovascular accident may also present with acute confusion; this may be misleading when neurological signs are unobtrusive. Metabolic causes include hypoglycaemic attacks, diabetic ketosis, uraemia and severe fluid or electrolyte disturbances. Myxoedema, pernicious anaemia and hypothermia may also produce acute delirium.

Drugs are another important cause. Multiple drug regimes are particularly likely to give trouble. Drugs acting on the central nervous system are most likely to be implicated. Perhaps most troublesome of these are the older drugs used in the treatment of Parkinson's disease such as benzhexol (Artane) and orphenadrine (Disipal). Of the newer anti-parkinsonian drugs, amantadine (Symmetrel) may occasionally give florid confusional states in which visual hallucinosis is a prominent feature whilst L-dopa is not completely trouble free although perhaps best of all the current drugs available in this respect. Tricyclic antidepressants such as imipramine, nortriptyline and amitriptyline are also quite potent causes of confusional states; undue agitation and restlessness often being a prominent feature. Sedatives, tranquillisers and anti-epileptic drugs may also precipitate confusional states. Barbiturate hypnotics have a particularly bad reputation amongst geriatricians in this regard.

Anaemia is often claimed to be an important cause of confusional states. Pernicious anaemia does appear to be important and heart failure secondary to anaemia may precipitate confusion. Apart from these possibilities, however, there is no clear evidence that anaemia itself is responsible (Hodkinson 1973).

Chronic confusion

Chronic confusion may occur when the physical cause of a confusional state is irreversible and persistent. Thus many old people may have prolonged confusion during their last illness. Chronic confusional states may often be seen in patients with intractable heart failure, hepatic failure, renal failure or terminal malignant disease. There may be persistent confusion after a massive cerebrovascular accident or in other continuing intracerebral lesions such as primary or secondary tumours of the brain or chronic subdural haematoma. One should remember some causes that, though rare, are potentially remediable. These include the reversible dementia associated with vitamin B_{12} deficiency, G.P.I. (now a considerable rarity) and 'communicating' or 'normal pressure' hydrocephalus (Bannister *et al.* 1967). This last can be recognised by isotope encephalography ('R.I.S.A. scan') and may be helped by drainage procedures. Myxoedema and chronic alcoholism are other possible diagnoses.

A substantial proportion of chronic confusion however is due to the dementing diseases for which we have no effective treatment; the main ones include senile dementia and arteriosclerotic or multi-infarct dementia. Parkinson's disease is fairly common in old age and may also be associated with progressive dementia. Parkinson's disease is now thought to have a degenerative rather than an arteriosclerotic basis.

Senile dementia

This is numerically the most important form of dementia, particularly in the older age groups and most especially in elderly women. Pathologically the histological changes in the brain, senile plaques and neurofibrillary tangles, are indistinguishable from those of Alzheimer's disease, a genetically determined pre-senile dementia. The clinical picture is a slowly progressive one spread over many years. Memory, especially recent memory, shows an early and conspicuous decline. As the disease progresses obvious disorientation and confusion become increasingly apparent. Restlessness, wandering and other behavioural disturbances tend to develop. The emotions become blunted and personal habits and cleanliness deteriorate. The patient becomes more and more unable to care for herself and may become incontinent of urine and later of faeces. Physical health is not affected until the very late stages of the disease when dementia is profound. Weight loss may then be considerable, mobility deteriorates and hypostatic pneumonia commonly terminates the illness.

Arteriosclerotic dementia

Arteriosclerotic dementia results from loss of brain tissue due to multiple infarcts and it seems that loss of 50 ml or more of brain tissue is required. Arteriosclerotic dementia affects males more than females and tends to occur at relatively earlier ages. The mental manifestations are indistinguishable from those of senile dementia except for differences in the time course of their development. Thus a slow and steady deterioration characterises senile dementia whereas deterioration in arteriosclerotic dementia is by a stepwise decline due to repeated infarctions. Distinction otherwise rests on the absence of C.N.S. signs in senile dementia and the finding of bilateral pyramidal signs in arteriosclerotic dementia. Other manifestations of arterial disease may also be found and hypertension may be associated with it. Prognosis is somewhat worse than in senile dementia as death may result from a major stroke, myocardial infarction or other vascular catastrophe.

Conditions mimicking chronic confusion

Other conditions may mimic chronic confusion. Pseudodementia occurring as a clinical variant of depressive illness needs to be distinguished as the prognosis with appropriate treatment is good. Occasionally dysphasia may give rise to diagnostic difficulty, particularly the 'jargon' form of dysphasia in which marked receptive difficulty prevents the monitoring of speech. The patient's speech then becomes a bizarre jumble of non-sequiturs, neologisms and disconnected words and phrases which can be mistaken for gross confusion due to dementia. Recognition of the dysphasic character of the speech and the history of sudden onset of the disability should prevent this mistake being made.

DEPRESSION AND APATHY

Depressive illness

Depressive illness is the commonest of the affective disorders and has an incidence which rises steadily with age. It has a strong tendency to recur, but in many old people depressive illness presents for the first time. Although genetic factors are involved in depressive illness, their operation is often less clearly seen in old age. Depression has been categorised into two main types, neurotic-reactive and psychotic-endogenous but this distinction is difficult to make in many elderly patients and does not seem to be therapeutically or prognostically important. However, reactive mechanisms can quite often be postulated in elderly patients with depression, bereavement, physical illness and social disabilities being common; but correction of such extrinsic factors may have little effect on the course of the illness.

Patients with depressive illness look and feel depressed. Insomnia, characterised by early waking rather than difficulty getting off to sleep, and anorexia are cardinal symptoms. There tends to be a reduction of general activity and slowness of speech and movement. Agitation may often be prominent but others show apathy and withdrawal which when extreme simulate dementia—the pseudodementia already referred to. Patients may complain of listlessness, lack of energy and feelings of guilt, unworthiness or uselessness. Hypochondriacal delusions may be prominent such as a belief that the bowels are blocked or that the organs are rotting inside the patient's body or there may be multiple aches and pains. Suicidal thoughts are common. These may amount to no more than vague feelings put into such a common remark as 'I wish the Lord would take me' but are often more compelling. Suicidal thoughts are certainly to be taken seriously in elderly depressed patients where the suicide risk is many times that in younger depressives. It is some four times greater in men than in women (Barraclough 1971). Those at risk of suicide are characterised by moderate depression with marked sleep disturbance and hypochondriacal symptoms. The depressive episode is usually of recent onset and is often the first attack and has usually already led to the enlistment of medical help. There is an association with serious physical illness and living alone.

The recognition of depressive illness is often far from straightforward, indeed it is probably the diagnosis that is most often missed in elderly patients. Those concerned with elderly patients need to think consciously of the possibility of depression all the time. Appetite and sleep disturbances should be the subject of routine enquiry and due regard should be paid to a depressed appearance. It is unwise to be too ready to assume that the patient can reasonably be expected to be a little miserable given the particular circumstances. A past history of depressive illness should put one on one's guard especially. Some people are hypochondriacal and valetudinarian all their lives but when such features arise for the first time in old age they strongly indicate depression. The role of drugs in the causation of depression should be remembered, reserpine and methyl dopa being the most commonly involved. Depression can also be a presentation of myxoedema.

Depressive symptoms in other diseases

Depressive symptoms or colouring may be a feature of other forms of mental illness. Depressive features in dementia can lead to diagnostic difficulties both because of the problems of distinguishing between true dementia and pseudodementia and because dementia and depression may not infrequently coexist—early dementia being an important trigger to depressive illness. A therapeutic trial of antidepressant therapy may be justifiable in order to resolve such diagnostic dilemmas.

Similarly, depressive symptoms may feature in paranoid psychoses and sometimes also in confusional states.

Self-willed death

This dramatic form of acute depressive reaction is occasionally seen in elderly patients and can best be described by illustration with an actual case history. An elderly lady in good health but severely disabled by arthritis required considerable support from relatives with whom she lived. She required considerable persuasion before she would agree to a fortnight's admission to hospital so that the relatives could take a holiday. When the time for her planned discharge arrived the relatives adamantly refused to accept her home again. Thereupon the patient literally turned her face to the wall and would barely speak, eat or drink. She died within two weeks.

Apathy

Apathy may be seen in a number of situations other than depressive illness. Lack of initiative and apathy are commonly found as features of dementia, adding to the difficulties of recognising whether or not depression might coexist. Some degree of apathy is also to be found in many chronically ill or disabled old people in whom it can also be difficult to decide whether there might not be a superadded depression. This is particularly so in the elderly in institutional care where it may be regarded as an aspect of institutionalisation but can be minimised by maintaining a proper atmosphere of liveliness and therapeutic activity.

AGITATION AND ANXIETY

Anxiety is a natural reaction to stress and may frequently occur, at any rate in mild form, in ill old people with good reason.

Morbid anxiety and agitation on the other hand may indicate psychiatric disturbances, particularly depressive illness although they may also occur in acute delirium, mania and dementia. In addition agitation and anxiety may be manifestations of physical conditions. Thyrotoxicosis is a classical example although only a minority of cases in old age show a typical clinical picture. The form of fearful agitation referred to as angor animi and classically associated with ischaemic heart disease may also sometimes be seen in other severe and mortal illnesses such as dissection of the aorta or left ventricular failure. Severe agitation may occur in hypoglycaemia, whether spontaneous or due to overtreatment, and also as a withdrawal symptom in patients habituated to alcohol or barbiturates. Drugs may also be responsible as for example the atropine-like tricyclic or anti-parkinsonian drugs; imipramine and benzhexol being particularly blameworthy. Sometimes sympatheticomimetic drugs such as ephedrine or saventerine may be responsible.

HALLUCINATIONS AND DELUSIONS

Hallucinations may sometimes be based on physical disease. Thus blind people may have visual hallucinations perhaps rather in the same way that phantom limb phenomena may persist after amputations. Drugs may also give hallucinosis, the hallucinations typically being visual as with benzhexol or atropine intoxication or in confusional states associated with amantadine treatment. Hallucinations may also be a feature of drug withdrawal as in delirium tremens of alcohol withdrawal. Temporal lobe epilepsy and narcolepsy are other rare causes.

More often hallucinations and delusions are a part of psychiatric illness. The common somatic delusions and delusions of guilt, unworthiness or poverty occurring in depression have already been mentioned. Hallucinations and delusions may also occur in acute or chronic confusion. The hallucinations of dementia are more often visual, the patient seeing vague figures of strangers or perhaps a dead relative with whom they may hold a conversation. Delusions are commonly that belongings, which they have lost because of poor memory, have been stolen.

Hallucinations in which a lost loved one is seen or heard are quite a common occurrence in the recently bereaved and should perhaps only be regarded as abnormal if they are unduly persistent.

PARANOID SYMPTOMS

Paranoid symptoms—hallucinations or delusions with a persecutory flavour, and paranoid behaviour—unwarranted suspiciousness—are typically due to paranoid psychosis, sometimes called senile paraphrenia. This schizophrenia-like condition occurs usually in old women who may have quite well preserved though eccentric personalities and who may manage to survive in the community surprisingly well, thanks perhaps to the tolerance of neighbours and police to whom they can be such a trial! They are usually socially isolated and a surprisingly high proportion have severe bilateral deafness (Cooper et al. 1974). Hallucinations are predominantly auditory and delusions may be well systematised. They may be helped by phenothiazine therapy which can be given as long-acting injections of fluphenazine where cooperation regarding oral therapy is likely to be poor.

Myxoedema may sometimes produce a paranoid psychosis, the 'myxoedematous madness' described by Richard Asher.

SELF-NEGLECT

Some old people seriously neglect themselves. They fail to keep themselves and their living accommodation clean, dress deteriorates, heating is inadequate and they do not feed themselves properly. They fail to seek medical attention even when it is obviously necessary and may refuse all forms of outside help. Where such self-neglect is long standing it may represent a lifelong personality disorder, marked eccentricity or senile paraphrenia. In such circumstances intellect may be well preserved, indeed there may be little overt psychiatric abnormality other than the self-neglect and this type of situation has been described as the senile squalor syndrome (McMilan & Shaw 1966) or the Diogenes syndrome (Clark *et al.* 1975). Other instances are due to long standing dementia.

When self-neglect is of more recent origin it may well be due to depression but may be due to physical disease. Chronic physical illness may lead to self-neglect because of an accompanying persistent confusional state or where there is marked apathy as for example in myxoedema. Sometimes, increasing physical disability in a person who had been too proud to accept timely outside help may lead to such a deterioration of standards that they are then too ashamed and demoralised to allow any interference.

ABNORMAL BEHAVIOUR

Wandering behaviour is a troublesome feature of both the dementias and acute confusional states and is particularly likely at night. Shouting and noisy behaviour occur under the same conditions. The paranoid behaviour of paraphrenics may disturb the peace of the neighbourhood. Aggressive behaviour may be a distressing occurrence in dements or in those with confusional states.

Alcoholism

Alcoholic addiction is not rare in old age. It may give rise to various forms of antisocial behaviour such as self-neglect, persistent drunkenness, noisiness or aggressiveness.

Sexual misdemeanours

Dementia or confusional states may lead to sexual disinhibition and minor misdemeanours such as exposure and stripping are not uncommon. Occasionally, confused old men may make persistent amorous advances to female staff or patients but these are more likely to be the cause of gentle amusement rather than serious concern! More serious sexual offences in old age are less likely to be due to such disinhibition from mental impairment. Old men charged with such offences are more often of normal intellect and personality. Their abnormal behaviour, which may involve sexually immature girls, often seems to be based on developing impotence which leads to attempts at gratification by incomplete sexual activities. They often seem to be men who have tended to overvalue themselves in terms of their sexual performance when younger.

Mania

Mania accounts for only a very small proportion of the affective disorders of old age, being dwarfed by the very high frequency of depression. It may give rise to considerable behaviour disturbance but tends to present a less fully developed and less typical picture than in younger adults. Fully fledged 'flight of ideas' is unusual, rather there is overactivity, garrulousness or meanderings of an anecdotal kind. Tense, unhappy and bewildered mood is more common than the classical euphoria, and delusions may be more paranoid, sexually oriented or of depressive cast than grandiose. The clinical picture may resemble that of acute delirium and be difficult to distinguish from it.

4

RHEUMATIC AND LOCOMOTOR SYMPTOMS

'RHEUMATISM'

'Rheumatism' is a vague term implying generalised stiffness, discomfort, aching or pain in muscles, bones or joints. There are many diagnostic possibilities, pathologies in the nervous system, muscles, bones or joints all needing to be taken into consideration.

Nervous system diseases which may lead to a complaint of rheumatism may do so by virtue of rigidity, spasticity, pain or paraesthesiae. Parkinson's disease is common but easy to overlook, as has already been pointed out. Rigidity is its chief manifestation but vague discomfort or aching may also occur. The characteristic facies, attitude and gait should draw attention to the diagnosis. Spasticity leading to a complaint of rheumatism may be due to pseudobulbar palsy, motor neurone disease, subacute combined degeneration of the cord or to cervical spondylosis with myelopathy. Peripheral neuritis, most often due to diabetes or carcinoma of the bronchus, may give rheumatism comprising paraesthesiae, weakness and clumsiness.

Muscular pain and stiffness may occur in febrile illness such as influenza. It is a particular feature of polymyalgia rheumatica. This is a manifestation of cranial arteritis which, though not particularly common, occurs especially in old age. It is most important to recognise the condition promptly and begin steroid therapy. This gives excellent relief but also prevents the development of the most serious complication of cranial arteritis, sudden blindness due to retinal artery occlusion. Polymyalgia rheumatica has an acute or subacute onset with generalised muscular aches and pains, morning stiffness and sometimes fever. The E.S.R. is usually considerably raised. There may be temporal headache and a tender, thickened temporal artery, biopsy of which will show the typical giant cell arteritis.

Muscular pain or discomfort may also be secondary to skeletal deformities such as kyphoscoliosis. It may also be ascribed to 'non-articular rheumatism' or 'fibrositis' but these terms have no pathological basis and are best avoided.

Rarely, muscular pain may be due to dermatomyositis or a polymyositis associated with collagen diseases such as systemic sclerosis or with malignant disease.

Bone pain may be the main presenting symptom in osteomalacia. This is a generalised disease of bone where the osteoid matrix fails to calcify adequately due to a lack of vitamin D. Skin synthesis of vitamin D relies on exposure to ultra-violet light and it is perhaps only when such exposure is insufficient or lacking that dietary intake of vitamin D becomes important (Hodkinson et al. 1973). Osteomalacia in old age thus occurs principally in the housebound, the generally poor dietary intake of vitamin D then becoming critical. It is also particularly likely to develop after gastrectomy or where there is a malabsorption syndrome. Occasionally it may accompany the protracted intake of barbiturate or anti-epileptic drugs which lead to enzyme induction in the liver and to the more rapid destruction of vitamin D by conversion to inactive metabolites. Apart from bone pain, patients with osteomalacia may have proximal muscle weakness producing a characteristic waddling gait. They are more likely to have fractures, particularly of the ribs. Radiology may show the pathognomonic Looser's zones, bands of radiolucency across bones and particularly occurring in scapulae, ribs, pubis or femora. Biochemical investigation typically shows hypocalcaemia, low phosphate and raised alkaline phosphatase.

Bone biopsy confirms the diagnosis, undecalcified sections showing excessive amounts of uncalcified osteoid.

Secondary deposits are another important cause of bone pain. These are most commonly from carcinoma of the prostate, breast or lung. Alternatively deposits may be due to multiple myelomatosis. Lytic deposits seen on skeletal X-rays are consistent with any of these diagnoses. Myeloma typically causes no elevation of alkaline phosphatase in contrast to the others and may also be distinguished by the very high globulin and a monoclonal band on electrophoresis. Sclerotic bony deposits indicate carcinoma of breast or prostate and in the latter case there may be a diagnostically elevated acid phosphatase. There should always be a careful examination of the potential primary sites; examination of the breasts and rectal examination should not be omitted in examination of elderly patients.

Paget's disease may involve widespread areas of the skeleton and the involved bones may sometimes be painful. The pain tends to have a boring or throbbing character. The characteristic radiological changes and raised alkaline phosphatase allow ready diagnosis.

Osteoporosis is a very common condition in old age but is not a cause of pain unless fractures occur.

Diseases of the joints must be considered next. Osteoarthritis is extremely common and usually presents little diagnostic difficulty. The main exception to this is when there are prominent Bouchard's nodes. These are equivalent to Heberden's nodes but occur at the proximal instead of terminal interphalangeal joints and may mislead those unacquainted with them to mistakenly diagnose rheumatoid arthritis.

Rheumatoid arthritis is rarely of recent onset. More usually it began in young adult life or middle age and has now reached a 'burnt out', clinically inactive stage with considerable secondary degenerative change. Joint changes may be gross, for example arthritis mutilans of the hands may quite often be present. Non-articular manifestations are also quite often seen, e.g. rheumatoid nodules, tendinopathy such as tenosynovial changes or tendon rupture, Sjögren's syndrome and severe generalised osteoporosis.

Other forms of polyarthritis such as ankylosing spondylitis, Reiter's syndrome, psoriatic arthropathy or the arthropathy of ulcerative colitis are seen occasionally but almost always are of long standing.

A rare arthropathy that may begin in old age is hypertrophic pulmonary osteoarthropathy. This consists of clubbing, periostitis at the wrists and ankles and polyarthritis and is an unusual manifestation of carcinoma of the bronchus.

Finally, one should remember the possibility that rheumatism may be an expression of hypochondriasis in depression or in psychoneurotic personalities.

BACK PAIN

Few individuals who reach old age have a spine which shows no pathological changes. The vast majority have either osteoporosis or osteoarthritis, but the two processes tend to be mutually exclusive, a severe degree of both osteoporosis and osteoarthritis rarely occurring together in the same individual. Osteoporosis is characterised by decreased radiological density of the vertebrae with often partial collapse as shown by a 'codfish vertebra' appearance or by more severe collapse with wedging. Clinically there may be evidence of loss of vertebral height such as an increased span to height ratio or a transverse abdominal skin crease. Osteoarthritis of the spine includes disc degeneration and narrowing, sclerosis of bone margins and osteophyte formation which may be gross.

Both these common pathologies may give rise to back pain but usually they do not; as they are such ubiquitous conditions it is unwise to attribute back pain, particularly if it is severe or a new complaint, to these causes too readily. It is amazing how few old people with spinal osteoporosis can be induced to admit to any significant backache. Osteoporosis tends to give severe back pain only when there has been recent trauma, perhaps resulting in acute vertebral collapse, when the osteoporosis is severe and rapidly progressive (and this is seldom met with in geriatric practice) or when steroid therapy has exacerbated the process. Osteoarthritis, though commonly resulting in stiffness of the back, often gives little or no pain. It may, however, give rise to acute low back pain, often with pain down the leg simulating the sciatica of a disc lesion, when the sacroiliac joint is also osteoarthritic and is subjected to minor trauma. The pain is typically worse on movement, especially turning movements such as turning to look round to the side or rear whilst seated. The diagnosis is confirmed by the finding of localised tenderness over the sacroiliac joint and treatment by local infiltration of hydrocortisone and local anaesthetic tends to give gratifyingly good results. Sacroiliac pain is very often misdiagnosed as prolapsed intravertebral disc but this latter diagnosis appears to be excessively rare in old age.

Thus if there is no story of recent trauma or steroid therapy and if localised sacroiliac tenderness is absent, severe back pain of recent origin is likely to be due to other causes. Most important among these is malignant disease with spinal deposits. Carcinoma of prostate or breast are by far the commonest causes and are particularly important as hormonal treatment may be of considerable help. Rectal examination, and examination of the breasts in the female are thus key parts to the physical examination of the elderly person complaining of backache. Other carcinomata may also be responsible, e.g. lung, rectum or stomach and multiple myelomatosis is another important possibility. Spinal X-rays will usually demonstrate deposits and in the case of breast and prostate these may be sclerotic rather than lytic. A very high E.S.R. is typically found in myeloma and a proportion of cases may show Bence Jones' proteinuria. A high alkaline phosphatase is usually found with carcinomatous spinal deposits and the acid phosphatase is typically raised with metastases from the prostate. Sometimes spinal deposits may give rise to a progressive paraplegia, indeed this is the commonest cause of paraplegia in the elderly.

Other disease may present as back pain occasionally. Paget's disease commonly affects vertebrae and is usually asymptomatic but may rarely give rise to considerable pain, particularly following trauma. It is important not to confuse Paget's disease with sclerotic spinal metastases for, apart from the radiological similarities, both give a high alkaline phosphatase. Herpes zoster may give girdle pain round to the back and may cause diagnostic confusion in the few days before the rash appears. Ankylosing spondylitis hardly ever begins in old age but cases survive into the geriatric age group and may have persistent back pain. Rare but important causes of back pain include osteomyelitis, tuberculosis of the spine, pancreatitis, penetrating gastric ulcer and aneurysm of the aorta. Osteomalacia may give back pain but usually only as a part of more generalised skeletal pain.

PAINFUL LIMBS

Osteoarthritis or rheumatoid arthritis as causes of limb pain present no diagnostic difficulties other than the danger of overlooking fracture which has already been referred to.

Pathological fractures due to myelomatosis or carcinomatosis and traumatic fractures are usually obvious also. However, incomplete fractures may occur occasionally in bowed Pagetic limb bones, multiple small transverse cracks appearing on the outer convexity, rather as may happen on bending an unripe banana, and these may give rise to considerable pain.

Diagnosis of pain on exertion in the arm as being anginal or in the leg as intermittent claudication will usually be very straightforward. Oddly neither of these occur nearly as commonly as one would expect when the high prevalences of ischaemic heart disease and peripheral vascular disease are considered. This may in part be due to altered pain mechanisms in old age but perhaps merely indicates that the elderly may have other disabilities which preclude them from reaching the necessary level of exertion.

Painful legs may sometimes result from peripheral neuropathy. The rarity of root pain from prolapsed intervertebral disc has already been commented on. Similarly brachalgia from cervical spondylosis is surprisingly uncommon despite the frequency of advanced degenerative changes in the cervical spine in old age. Causalgia due to involvement of the brachial plexus by an apical carcinoma of bronchus is met with infrequently. Another occasional cause of pain in the arm is the shoulder–hand syndrome, a form of reflex dystrophy which may occur in association with hemiplegia, myocardial infarction or cervical spondylosis or without an obvious precipitating cause. There is painful atrophy, and contracture of the hand and patchy osteoporosis is seen on X-ray. This diagnosis should not be too readily made in the hemiplegic, unrecognised subluxation of the shoulder being a far more common reason for pain down the arm (Fitzgerald-Finch & Gibson 1975).

CRAMP

Night cramps in the legs is not a rare complaint of old people. Very occasionally it can be blamed on some recognised metabolic abnormality such as uraemia or hypocalcaemia but the vast majority defy rational explanation! However, the patients may often be helped by empirical therapy with quinine sulphate.

True tetany is uncommon, sometimes occurring as a result of hyperventilation in anxious patients and sometimes due to profound hypocalcaemia in osteomalacia. It is rather surprising that tetany is not seen more often in view of the considerable incidence of hypocalcaemia in ill old people.

Complaints of leg cramp attributable to intermittent claudication or the flexor spasms of paraplegia are other possibilities.

ACUTE JOINT PAIN

Acute joint pain may develop in a joint already the obvious site of osteoarthritis or rheumatoid arthritis. Acute exacerabation of an oestoarthritic joint is usually due to trauma, loose bodies formed by the detachment of osteophytes often being implicated. Exacerbation of a rheumatoid joint may represent a recrudescence of clinical activity of the disease. However, in either case one should bear in mind the possibility of superadded septic arthritis. This is none too rare an occurrence and infection is haematogenous, a further reminder that bacteraemia may quite often arise in ill old people. It is therefore wise practice to aspirate any arthritic joint which becomes acutely inflamed with signs of effusion.

Gout is another important cause of acute painful joints. In old age, females are quite likely to be affected. Diagnosis is usually straightforward when typical podagra occurs and when tophi are present. Thiazide diuretics are a provocative factor in quite a number of cases. Occasionally diagnostic mistakes are made when other joints are affected and there is marked surrounding soft tissue inflammation mistaken for a cellulitic infection. Diagnosis of gout is confirmed by the finding of a raised serum uric acid and typical punched out bone erosions on X-ray.

Pseudogout or calcium gout is less common than true gout but may be confused with it. The clinical picture is similar but in this case the arthritis is in response to deposition of crystals of calcium pyrophosphate within the joint instead of monosodium urate. The diagnosis is confirmed by demonstration of these positively birefringent crystals in the aspirated joint fluid but is also suggested when radiology shows articular cartilage calcification or calcification of the menisci of the knee. However, such calcifications are not rare in asymptomatic elderly subjects.

ABNORMALITIES OF GAIT

Abnormalities of gait may arise in a number of ways and these are classified in a rough and ready way below under the headings of deformity, pain, stiffness, weakness, ataxia and incoordination and involuntary movements. More than one of these physical mechanisms may operate in the individual case and psychological mechanisms may also be relevant. For example one may sometimes see a hysterical gait characterised by terrifying and dramatic lurching and staggering suggesting the grossest ataxia yet somehow the patient never quite falls down on the floor although he may subside safely on a bed or chair or pitch histrionically into the arms of the bystander.

Patients who have lost confidence in their balance may adopt a wide-based gait and hang on to furniture or people around them.

Deformity

Gait abnormalities due to deformities usually present no diagnostic difficulties. Abnormal gait and posture may draw attention to spinal deformities such as kyphosis or scoliosis. Shortening of a leg due to old fracture, Girdlestone operation or severe osteoarthritis of hip with gliding of the acetabulum up the ilium produce a dipping, 'dot and carry' gait. Bilateral osteoarthritis of hips may produce scissors gait or bizarre gaits where one grossly externally rotated leg leads and the other follows behind it. Gross disorganisation of knees due to advanced osteoarthritis or, uncommonly, Charcot's joint leading to lateral instability may give an unsteady wobbling gait where the affected knee stabilises itself in knock-kneed apposition to its healthy fellow. Unusual gait may also draw attention to bowing of legs due to childhood rickets or Paget's disease of tibia or femur.

Pain

Intermittent claudication, in other words intermittent limping, is a somewhat special case of pain leading to an abnormal gait. Painful feet due to corns, calluses, bunions, ulcers or ill-fitting shoes give a hobbling gait. Painful joints due to gout, osteo-arthritis or rheumatoid arthritis may have a similar effect. Limping may occasionally be due to bone pain from Paget's disease, secondary deposits, osteomalacia or undiagnosed fracture.

Stiffness

Stiffness may be of the joints or of the muscles. Very limited hip movements due to severe osteoarthritis may give a gait where progress is achieved by small lateral rocking movements, rather like walking a pair of protractors. Circumduction may result from a stiff knee.

Muscle stiffness is a feature of the gait abnormalities in hemiplegia and paraplegia and Parkinson's disease. The hemiplegic with marked spasticity of adductor muscles of the thigh shows a tendency to scissoring, the hemiplegic leg crossing in front of the good leg and the foot failing to make contact with the ground. Patients may correct for this hazard by adopting a crab-wise gait, walking sideways good leg first with the hemiplegic leg trailing so that friction against the floor prevents adduction. Bilateral spasticity as in a paraparesis leads to a tendency to drag the feet and to trip easily.

Parkinsonism produces very characteristic gait abnormalities with marche à petit pas, festinant gait, reduced arm swing and an attitude of flexion as common features.

Weakness

Proximal muscle weakness such as may develop in osteomalacia gives rise to a waddling gait. Distal muscle weakness results in foot drop and a high stepping gait as in peripheral neuritis. The combination of spasticity with foot drop in the hemiplegic limb produces the characteristic hemiplegic gait where the leg is circumducted to counteract the difficulties of bending the knee and clearing the foot.

Ataxia and incoordination

Unsteadiness of gait may occasionally be due to cerebellar ataxia as in multiple sclerosis surviving into the geriatric age group, to the sensory ataxia of peripheral neuritis or subacute combined degeneration of the cord or rarely to tabes dorsalis, usually an old treated case with persistent signs. Much more commonly incoordination is not due to such clearcut neurological entities but occurs in association with diffuse cerebral damage in demented elderly people. Geriatricians are familiar with a syndrome which is not to be found in neurological textbooks but is to be seen in most geriatric wards. Its characteristic features are the combination of a wide based gait showing marche à petit pas with a marked tendency to backward leaning. A more subtle feature is that the toes fail to grip as the patient walks but point upwards rather like a permanent Babinski sign. Though patients with this syndrome may have pyramidal or extrapyramidal signs, such signs may equally well be absent. Anxiety and a period of bed rest or inactivity may make matters worse but the association with mental impairment is so strong that a true neurological basis seems likely.

Involuntary movements

Sometimes, involuntary movements may affect gait. This is particularly likely in those with chorea or choreoathetosis. Mild chorea, often associated with some minor intellectual impairment, is quite common. Its aetiology is uncertain and it is usually termed senile chorea though a proportion of cases have an acute onset indicating a vascular cause. Chorea may also occur after treatment with phenothiazine tranquillisers but usually affects only the face as a facial dyskinesia characterised by spasmodic grimacing movements.

Very occasionally one sees hemiplegia with gross spasticity in which contact of the foot with the ground stimulates the onset of clonus. This can grossly affect the gait and render walking hazardous if the clonus is marked, the jerking movements tending to throw the patient off balance.

Creaking gait

Patients with severe osteoarthritis or rheumatoid arthritis with secondary degenerative changes may have marked joint crepitus that can be plainly heard by bystanders. The noise may be creaking, chirruping or cracking in quality and can be a considerable embarrassment to the unfortunate patient. Knees and hips are the most frequent source of these sounds although weight-bearing shoulder joints may be responsible in those walking with sticks or frames.

5

FALLS, FAINTS AND TURNS

FALLING ABOUT

Many old people have multiple falls, indeed 'falling about' is quite a common reason for referral for hospital admission. Females are particularly vulnerable; they not only have more falls but are more likely to sustain fractures when they do fall, presumably because they are more often osteoporotic.

The increased tendency to fall with age in part reflects a general tendency for the finer control of posture and balance to deteriorate in common with similar declines in many other physiological mechanisms (Overstall 1978). A considerable proportion of isolated single falls appear to be truly accidental but where falls are multiple, pathological mechanisms are often operating. Episodic impairments of balance may be responsible and these are discussed in the next section on giddiness. Transient loss of consciousness may present as falls and this will be dealt with in a later section on 'queer turns'.

Premonitory falls

A series of falls may herald the onset of an acute episode of illness. Such premonitory falls may thus be the first indication of a great variety of illnesses causing constitutional upset such as chest infections or heart failure. This is particularly likely in the very old and the more frail. Stroke may have an insidious onset over several days, the so-called ingravescent stroke, and several falls may occur before the hemiplegic weakness becomes obvious. Other causes of neurological weakness with an insidious onset may similarly present as falls whilst signs are minimal. Peripheral neuritis and paraparesis are examples.

Mental alertness

Many old people who do not fall avoid falling only because they take great care. Those with mental impairment fail to take as much care and fall very commonly. Thus admission to hospital with fracture of the femur is often the first presentation of an elderly dementing person to the hospital services. Dementia or acute confusional states may often be first brought to the attention of the general practitioner because relatives or neighbours have become concerned because of the tendency to fall.

The role of sedation should be remembered. Most night sedatives leave the old person with a hangover the following morning when diminished alertness and ataxia may result in falls. Daytime sedation with tranquillisers may present similar risks. The sedative effects of anti-epileptic drugs may also be hazardous, particularly in the case of epanutin which may also give quite marked ataxia in old people. Alcohol also deserves mention.

Liability to trip

An increased tendency to trip may result from abnormal gait (see p. 43), especially from small pace and shuffling gaits. Unsatisfactory footwear may also be a hazard as in the 'soft shoe shuffle' of those who wear oversize slippers.

Poor vision makes tripping more likely as obstacles are not seen. Old people often like a great deal of clutter in their homes and mats, rugs and other hazards combined with poor vision or miserliness over adequate lighting of the house may cause problems.

Other disabilities may impose sudden postural threats. Thus chorea, athetosis, spontaneous clonus or the sudden giving way of an unstable arthritic knee may result in falls. Sensory or motor ataxias may similarly be responsible.

Inability to regain balance

Normal people seldom fall because when their posture is threatened by a sudden trip they are usually able to quickly regain balance. For example, loss of balance forwards tends to be righted rapidly by throwing forwards the hips and trunk whilst head and neck are withdrawn backwards. This calls for flexibility of the hips and spine as well as an intact nervous system. Ability to regain balance is therefore compromised by arthritis of the hips, by stiffness or kyphosis of the thoraco-lumbar spine or by severe cervical spondylosis.

Parkinson's disease

Parkinsonism is a very important cause of liability to falls. The abnormalities of gait favour tripping whilst the rigidity, bradykinesis and attitude of flexion all conspire to make it virtually impossible for the unfortunate sufferer to regain balance once it has been at all seriously disturbed. Falls are not only common and frequent but often very heavy, particularly when the fall is to the rear. Parkinsonian patients may become afraid to walk without help because they are so terrified of falls. L-dopa therapy may lead to a dramatic improvement in this situation.

GIDDINESS

When a young patient complains of giddiness he can usually give a fairly clear account of the symptom which most usually consists of a true vertigo with a sense of rotation of the head or of the outside world. When an old person complains of giddiness or dizziness he is often far less clear as to what he means and when pressed as to details commonly proves not to have vertigo but rather a vague feeling of disordered spatial orientation, of feeling insecure or of being afraid of falling.

Often it may represent little more than a loss of confidence, perhaps following a number of falls or deterioration in mobility, coupled with the generally poorer balancing ability of the old. In some cases one suspects that some manipulative old people have found the complaint of giddiness to be a convenient way to get out of doing things they do not want to do and of gaining sympathy and attention. In other anxious old people or in those who are depressed it may be a more genuine psychogenic symptom. Oversedation may be responsible whilst other sorts of drug side effect may play a part, for example postural hypotension from anti-hypertensive drugs, the parkinsonian side effects of phenothiazines or the toxic effect of salicylates.

Abnormalities of gait, painful feet, general frailty or lateral instability of knees may engender feelings of insecurity whilst the serious loss of confidence in Parkinson's disease has already been stressed.

Giddiness may be a presenting symptom of anaemia or of recent bleeding. Faintness and giddiness may occur in shocked patients who are hypotensive. Postural hypotension, more fully considered in the next section, may also be responsible. In contrast, hypertension should not be accepted as an explanation of giddiness except perhaps in malignant hypertension and this is excessively rare in old age. When hypertensive patients do complain of giddiness it is either unrelated to their blood pressure or is an anxiety symptom due to their being aware and fearful of the diagnosis.

Ear disease, most commonly the blocking of the auditory meatus by wax, may give vertigo. Streptomycin may give rise to permanent vestibular damage in the elderly and should not be used where alternative drugs are available. Vertigo may occur as an acute disturbance in thrombosis of the posterior inferior cerebellar artery, with raised intracranial pressure or as a presenting symptom of an acoustic neuroma but all these situations are uncommon.

QUEER TURNS

Patients may complain of 'attacks', 'blackouts', 'wee turns', fainting or fits, but there is often little distinction between the terms used and they can all be considered together under the usefully non-committal heading of 'queer turns'.

It may be very difficult to get a clear story of the queer turn as the patient may have no recollection of it and onlookers may be far from clear as to what precisely took place.

Epilepsy

This is one important possibility. Epilepsy is quite common in old age (*British Medical Journal* 1975) and is usually of grand mal type, petit mal being uncommon. However, Jacksonian fits or temporal lobe epilepsy may sometimes be encountered. The recent onset of epilepsy in old age may often call for full investigation and may prove to be due to meningioma, glioma or other intracerebral disease. However, epilepsy may occur following stroke (Fine 1967). Metabolic causes of fits such as hypoglycaemia also need to be considered and fits may also occur during Stokes Adams attacks. Epileptiform convulsions may also herald the onset of a cerebrovascular accident.

Postural hypotension

Postural hypotension is a common reason for queer turns. As the name implies, the attacks usually occur when the patient first stands up from sitting. However, postural hypotension is more likely to be overlooked in the minority of patients in whom hypotension only develops after walking a little way, the exercise being necessary to the full development of the episode. Whenever there is any suspicion of postural hypotension it should be tested for by recording blood pressure in recumbency and then with the patient standing for some time. A fall of 20 mm Hg or more is usually taken as postural hypotension but patients with symptoms due to postural hypotension often show much greater falls than this. The homoeostatic control of blood pressure is less efficient in old people (Exton-Smith 1978), however postural hypotension in the elderly is usually attributable to some provocative factor such as hyponatraemia, anaemia or the toxic effects of drugs. It is also far more likely where there is evidence of cerebral damage, for example in those with stroke. The drugs most often responsible are the anti-hypertensive ganglion blocking drugs which are often given to elderly patients for quite inadequate reasons. The phenothiazine tranquillisers and the tricyclic antidepressants also have the ability to precipitate attacks of postural hypotension. Diuretics may be responsible when they lead to hyponatraemia.

Syncope

Ordinary fainting attacks can occur in the old much as in the young. They may be an early indication of the onset of constitutional illness and are also facilitated by anaemia. Often, however, apparent faints may represent cardiovascular disturbances of a more serious kind such as dysrhythmias, small pulmonary emboli, myocardial infarction or more rarely carotid sinus syndrome. Rhythm disturbances have been claimed to account for a substantial proportion of queer turns resulting in falls (Livesley & Atkinson 1974). Stokes Adams attacks are not rare and are due to a period of asystole usually at the time of a change from partial to complete heart block and tend not to occur once complete heart block has become established. Less severe syncope may accompany other rhythm changes such as the transition from sinus rhythm to atrial fibrillation or can occur during paroxysmal tachycardias. Syncope is not a particularly usual manifestation of aortic stenosis in old age.

Pulmonary embolism may not rarely present with nothing more than a brief queer turn. A series of such minor syncopal attacks due to a succession of small emboli may be far from benign however, and lead to marked, if non-specific, deterioration and death. The true cause may only be recognised at autopsy unless use is made of radio-fibrinogen screening for thromboembolism in specially at risk patients such as those with recent stroke (Denham et al. 1973).

Two uncommon causes of syncope are micturition syncope and defaecation syncope (Pathy 1977). These rather similar syndromes consist of syncope immediately following emptying of the bladder or rectum, particularly at night. Reflex hypotension appears to be responsible.

Cerebrovascular disease

Transient ischaemic attacks or 'little strokes' are sometimes seen but have tended to be overdiagnosed. The same is true of vertebro-basilar insufficiency and of internal carotid insufficiency; both undeniably occur in the elderly, giving rise to transient attacks of disturbance of consciousness and various neurological deficits, but undoubted cases are rare.

'Drop-attacks'

Drop-attacks have tended to be accorded a special place in geriatric medicine ever since they were described with such persuasive brilliance by Sheldon (1960). He ascribed a quarter of falls in an elderly series to this cause. He suggested that drop-attacks, sudden falls occurring without any warning and without loss of consciousness, were a specific entity and had as a further characteristic a peculiar form of difficulty in getting up from the ground again due to a temporary loss of muscle tone which reverted to normal once the victim had been stood up again. However, many old people have difficulty getting up from the ground for perfectly mundane reasons (Hodkinson 1962). It now seems very doubtful that drop-attacks represent any genuine pathological entity. Recent work (Stevens & Matthews 1973) has indicated that drop-attacks, defined in the study as 'falling without warning, not apparently due to any malfunction of the legs, not induced by change of posture or movement of the head, and not accompanied by vertigo or other cephalic sensation', occur almost entirely in women and often start in middle life. They appear to occur only whilst walking and appear most likely to be due to some feature of the female gait and not to any neurological or cardiovascular abnormality.

Other causes

Queer turns may sometimes represent brief acute episodes of left ventricular failure. Hypoglycaemia occurring as a spontaneous phenomenon in islet cell tumour may also present in this way. Rare causes are hysterical overbreathing leading to tetany and light headedness and the occurrence of occulogyric crises in post-encephalitic parkinsonism.

DROWSINESS, STUPOR AND COMA

Here we are concerned with more prolonged episodes of disturbance of consciousness than have already been dealt with under the heading of queer turns. Disturbed consciousness may occur in almost any episode of severe illness and is particularly common in terminal illness of any cause. Acute confusional states may quite often show some drowsiness and may go into stupor or coma as the medical condition worsens. More sudden onset of disturbance of consciousness may be seen with massive pulmonary embolism or myocardial infarction. This may be contrasted with a more gradual decline of consciousness with overwhelming infections, hypostatic pneumonia, septicaemia or severe cardiac failure for example. Major abdominal catastrophes may similarly present with nothing other than malaise and deteriorating consciousness. Thus, the perforation of a peptic ulcer or a mesenteric embolism may present in this way.

Intoxications

Disturbed consciousness may be due to metabolic intoxications as in uraemia, liver failure or carbon dioxide narcosis in respiratory disease. Drug intoxications are also important. These may be due to an intentional overdose, most commonly of barbiturate or other hypnotics, the high suicide risk of depression in old age having been commented on earlier. More often, however, injudicious therapy is to blame. Too great a dose of a hypnotic with consequent hangover or overenthusiastic dosage of tranquillisers or sedatives are met commonly. The diazepine tranquillisers may produce extreme drowsiness or even coma in quite small doses in some old people who appear to have abnormal sensitivity to them. Quite usual doses of sedatives may also give rise to disproportionately great sedation in certain illnesses, for example in pernicious anaemia (Cantor 1963) or after myocardial infarction where chlorpromazine in modest doses may devastatingly oversedate. The sedative side effects of drugs given for other reasons should be remembered, for example anti-epileptic drugs, antihistamines, some of the tricyclic antidepressants and the more potent analgesics. Overindulging in alcohol may also be to blame.

Neurological disorders

Disturbance of consciousness is a common feature of the presentation of cerebrovascular accidents. Very sudden onset suggests cerebral embolism, rapidly deteriorating consciousness cerebral haemorrhage, whereas the disturbance is more slowly developing in cerebral thrombosis, indeed often does not occur. Fluctuating drowsiness is particularly suggestive of subdural haematoma, particularly where there is a story of a recent fall or other trauma to the head. More rarely disturbed consciousness may be due to primary or secondary cerebral tumour, to cerebral abscess or, very rarely, to encephalitis. There may be a fairly prolonged period of drowsiness after an epileptic fit whilst narcolepsy may be seen very occasionally.

Disturbance of consciousness in the diabetic patient

Cerebrovascular accident is probably the commonest cause of a disturbance of consciousness in the elderly diabetic patient. However, alternative possibilities are the occurrence of hypoglycaemia when the dose of either insulin or oral agent is too great, or the onset of diabetic pre-coma or coma. Diabetic ketotic pre-coma and coma are far from rare and may well occur in what has hitherto been regarded as a mild case, perhaps treated only by dietary regulation. Intercurrent infection may be responsible for triggering the attack. Hyperosmolar non-ketotic diabetic coma is seen from time to time. Here, enormously high blood sugars are found without there being any ketosis. Mortality is high, especially if not recognised and treated promptly. A pitfall is that transient hemiparesis may occur and this may lead to misdiagnosis as stroke. Drowsiness in a diabetic should always lead to prompt determination of the blood sugar.

Other causes

Hypothermia of any severity almost invariably results in drowsiness or coma. The diagnosis is far less likely to be missed if one is familiar with the characteristic clinical picture. The patient is drowsy and confused and has a waxy and pale appearance often strongly reminiscent of myxoedema. There is no shivering or complaint of feeling cold but the abdomen feels cold to the examining hand. Tendon reflexes show delay of relaxation identical to the 'hung-up' reflexes found in myxoedema. Diagnosis is confirmed by a five-minute rectal thermometer temperature of 35°C or less. Bradycardia is usual and may be marked with more severe degrees of hypothermia. Hypothermia is often secondary to severe physical disease but a minority of cases are due to myxoedema. Phenothiazine tranquillisers predispose to hypothermia as they inhibit shivering. Mortality of hypothermia is high though this is perhaps largely an expression of the strong association with severe illness which may often have a very poor prognosis in its own right.

Myxoedema is an unusual but important cause of coma in old age (Impallomeni 1977). It is often accompanied by generalised convulsions and may be preceded by headache. The hypothyroidism is usually profound.

Coma due to Simmonds' disease or hypertensive encephalopathy is of extreme rarity in old age.

Finally, one may occasionally see hysterical or feigned unconsciousness in psychoneurotic or manipulative old people.

6

CARDIO-RESPIRATORY PRESENTATIONS

SWOLLEN LEGS

Leg oedema is very common in the elderly, particularly in women. Its presence is often far too readily assumed to be due to cardiac failure and diuretics may then be prescribed unnecessarily. A survey of patients admitted to a geriatric department showed that 34% had been receiving diuretics from their general practitioner! Cardiac failure is, of course, a major reason for the development of leg oedema in old people but should not be diagnosed unless there are other confirmatory signs such as sacral oedema, basal crepitations, liver engorgement and elevation of jugular venous pressure.

Not all swollen legs represent oedema; some are due to lymphoedema rather than pitting oedema, whilst some fat ladies have very thick ankles due solely to fat. Let us look further at some of the alternative causes of true leg oedema.

Venous disease

Varicose veins are commonplace and may often be accompanied by ankle oedema. Many patients may have had an old venous thrombosis giving rise to persistent leg oedema whilst the recent onset of oedema of the leg may indicate a new deep vein thrombosis. Deep venous thrombosis is particularly common in immobile elderly patients who are acutely ill. It is particularly likely to occur after stroke or myocardial infarction. Homan's sign, pain in the calf when the foot is dorsiflexed, is not always present but is none the less a useful confirmatory sign.

Occasionally more proximal venous compression or occlusion may be responsible for leg oedema, e.g. occlusion of the pelvic veins or inferior vena cava obstruction or compression by ascites or tumour.

The association of venous thrombosis with malignant disease, especially carcinoma of the pancreas, should be remembered when multiple thromboses are seen.

Immobility

Immobility can lead to leg oedema because the normal muscular pumping action assisting venous return is lacking. Old people who spend most of the day sitting in a chair often have a little oedema of the ankles. More marked oedema is common in arthritic patients, especially those with rheumatoid arthritis. This is particularly likely when there is effusion into the knee joint adding an element of venous obstruction. Quite considerable oedema is commonly found in the hemiplegic limb, similarly leg oedema is often found for some time after fracture of the femur.

Mechanical oedema may also result from the garters worn by some old ladies or from the common alternative of twisting the stocking top to keep it up.

Generalised fluid retention

Leg oedema may be seen as a part of more generalised fluid retention in uraemia, cirrhosis, severe hypoproteinaemia or rarely in constrictive pericarditis. Fluid retention is an important side effect of some drugs. Chief among these is stilboestrol, often given in high dosage for carcinoma of breast or prostate in elderly patients, which commonly gives considerable fluid retention and may precipitate frank cardiac failure. Phenylbutazone, biogastrone and corticosteroids are other quite commonly used drugs which are similarly liable to result in sodium retention and the development of leg oedema.

Causes of cardiac failure

When leg oedema is due to cardiac failure, the aetiology of this is often difficult to ascertain with certainty, Pomerance (1972) having shown by her pathological studies that many minor pathologies may be acting in combination in such cases. However, in other patients the causation may be more straightforward. Ischaemic heart disease is quite common and cardiac failure may often be the mode of presentation where there has been a silent myocardial infarction. Valvular disease is also frequent. Mitral incompetence is most commonly the cause of a systolic murmur, although aortic stenosis or sclerosis are quite common. It is not rare for calcified valves to be visible on chest radiographs. Though far less common than incompetence, mitral stenosis is also seen and there are occasional instances of aortic incompetence. Hypertension is seldom severe enough to be the sole cause of heart failure but may be a contributory factor in some patients. Classical cor pulmonale due to severe emphysema is rare but acute cor pulmonale may follow pulmonary embolism and acute chest infections very commonly precipitate cardiac failure. Change of heart rhythm, particularly the onset of tachycardia or atrial fibrillation may also lead to cardiac failure. Thyrotoxicosis commonly presents with cardiac failure in old age but may be otherwise atypical and difficult to recognise clinically. Routine screening tests are necessary if the diagnosis is not to be missed. Anaemia and the development of subacute bacterial endocarditis are further possible precipitants of heart failure.

Cardiac amyloidosis deserves brief mention. Amyloidosis may occur principally or solely in the heart and its incidence rises with age so that the majority of those within the tenth decade may show some degree of cardiac amyloidosis (Pomerance 1966). Recent work suggests that even modest grades of cardiac amyloidosis may result in cardiac failure or contribute to it in combination with other minor pathological changes (Hodkinson & Pomerance 1977). Senile cardiac amyloidosis seems to be a type of primary amyloidosis with no recognisable precipitating factors and cannot be diagnosed in life at the present time.

SHORTNESS OF BREATH

Shortness of breath is a very important complaint in old age. It is a common disability, so much so that many old people may accept dyspnoea as 'normal' for their age and not complain of it but rather be seen to be breathless by the doctor or relatives. Shortness of breath may be noticed only as a slight increase in respiratory rate but can be a most important diagnostic observation in an unwell old person as it may be the only clinical clue to the diagnosis of pneumonia, heart failure or pulmonary embolism for example.

In view of the very many possible causes of shortness of breath it is useful to consider these under four broad subdivisions of the symptom; shortness of breath at rest, shortness of breath on exertion, orthopnoea and shortness of breath brought on by a change in posture.

Shortness of breath at rest

The sudden onset of dyspnoea at rest suggests pulmonary embolism, myocardial infarction or paroxysmal tachycardia as the most probable diagnoses. A rarer cause of sudden dyspnoea is spontaneous pneumothorax, perhaps less common than might be anticipated because so many old people have pleural adhesions as a result of lung disease in their earlier life. A subacute onset of dyspnoea may be due to many causes. Respiratory infections and heart failure rank as the most common among these.

Pneumonia, whether lobar pneumonia, bronchopneumonia, aspiration or hypostatic pneumonia, may present without fever or cough and with shortness of breath as the only specific symptom. An exacerbation of chronic bronchitis or attack of bronchial asthma are further possibilities, particularly when dyspnoea at rest arises against a background of chronic exertional dyspnoea. Metabolic disturbances may also produce shortness of breath at rest, for example the acidotic respiration of uraemia consisting of deep and rapid respiration (Küssmaul breathing) or that of diabetic ketosis. Rather more insidious onset of breathlessness may indicate the development of pleural effusion due to chronic heart failure, malignancy, 'synpneumonic' effusion developing in association with a pneumonia, pulmonary embolism or occasionally as a manifestation of rheumatoid arthritis. The less common but important possibility of an empyema should be remembered. Carcinoma of bronchus is another important cause, the development of dyspnoea being due to collapse, secondary obstructive pneumonia, large size of the tumour mass or metastases. Widespread pulmonary metastases from other primary sites may be responsible, carcinomatosis producing very severe dyspnoea when lymphangitis carcinomatosa occurs. Occasionally subacute onset of dyspnoea may be due to muscle weakness. In the elderly this is sometimes caused by motor neurone disease or peripheral neuropathies. Long-standing dyspnoea at rest is most commonly due to chronic bronchitis and emphysema.

Shortness of breath on exertion

Those diseases which may give dyspnoea at rest may, in less severe cases, give dyspnoea only on exertion. Dyspnoea on exertion is a typical manifestation of anaemia. Obesity is another important cause. Obesity is not so often seen in elderly men but is very common in old women. Other mechanical disabilities may also lead to exertional dyspnoea. An extreme example is the bilateral amputee walking on 'rocker' pylons where walking is achieved only by enormous muscular efforts so that exertional dyspnoea is common. Similarly grossly arthritic patients may become dyspnoeic. Ankylosing spondylitis is a special case however as chest cage movements are also much restricted by the disease. Severe kyphoscoliosis or chest deformities may act similarly.

Chronic structural lung disease such as emphysema, chronic interstitial pulmonary fibrosis, or old fibrocaseous pulmonary tuberculosis may give exertional breathlessness. Chronic interstitial pulmonary fibrosis, 'chronic Hamman-Rich syndrome', is most often seen in association with seropostive rheumatoid arthritis but also seems to occur in association with myxoedema. Occasional cases of occupational pulmonary fibrosis may be seen in old men.

Orthopnoea

Orthopnoea, shortness of breath brought on by lying flat, is typical of left ventricular failure and of the pulmonary oedema of mitral stenosis. The patient is typically woken from sleep by severe dyspnoea, so called paroxysmal nocturnal dyspnoea.

Postural dyspnoea

The common occurrence of orthopnoea neeeds to be distinguished from the occasional case where dyspnoea is dependent on posture and is due to mediastinal obstruction from a retrosternal goitre or from superior vena caval obstruction by malignant disease. This last syndrome is most often due to carcinoma of the bronchus involving mediastinal structures and impeding venous return from the head, neck and arms which show oedema and plethora. In addition, very unpleasant choking dyspnoea may be present which may be exacerbated by changes in neck position. Radiotherapy or chemotherapy with cytotoxic agents may give excellent symptomatic relief though they are only palliative.

Cheyne–Stokes respiration

Cheyne–Stokes respiration, when alternating periods of apnoea or hypopnoea and hyperpnoea occur, is quite common in severely ill old people, especially those with severe pulmonary oedema. When seen in the hyperpnoeic phase of the cycle it may be mistaken for other types of shortness of breath. Cheyne–Stokes breathing has always been regarded as having a most serious prognostic significance. However, in old age, it is a matter of some surprise how often patients showing this abnormality may make a recovery.

Psychogenic breathlessness

One may sometimes meet florid examples of hysterical overventilation, some episodes so severe that tetany may result. Very anxious patients may show less extreme psychogenic dyspnoea. Most commonly of all, however, are patients with some organic cause of breathlessness who become more breathless when they are more anxious. The patient with mild dyspnoea who becomes severely breathless during the ward round is commonplace—in some cases one feels that this psychological overlay of the symptom of dyspnoea comes very close to deliberate malingering in order to prolong stay in hospital!

Diagnosis of dyspnoea

Despite the many possible causes of breathlessness, diagnosis frequently presents few problems provided full use is made of the past history, of the history of the development and the type of dyspnoea and of the presence of associated symptoms such as wheeze, cough, expectoration or chest pain. Physical signs such as added sounds, dullness and altered breath sounds in the chest, tracheal shift, oedema and elevation of venous pressure may make diagnosis obvious. The chest X-ray is of the greatest value, often being clearly diagnostic. Electrocardiography and enzyme determinations may be helpful when cardiac pathology is responsible. Two situations present particular diagnostic difficulties, however. The first is the very frequent difficulty in distinguishing patchy bronchopneumonia from pulmonary oedema both clinically and radiologically and it is often concluded that both may be present together and treatment with both diuretics and antibiotics instituted to cover both possibilities. Secondly the diagnosis of pulmonary embolism is often difficult; indeed post-mortem examinations show time and again that the diagnosis has been missed in life. Only a minority of emboli produce any radiological change and many occur without there being any clinically obvious deep vein thrombosis present. Only the frequent utilisation of radiofibrinogen screening for thromboembolism can hope to improve the recognition of this frequent complication of illness in old age.

CHEST PAIN

Though old people less often complain of pain, chest pain none the less remains an important presenting symptom of disease in the age group. Pain may originate from the chest wall or spine, from the trachea, lungs or pleura, from the heart and great vessels, from gastrointestinal structures or may be psychogenic.

Pain originating from the chest wall and spine

Pain from bony structures is common. Fractures of the ribs are frequent. These may be cough fractures, a result of falls or may be secondary to either osteomalacia or osteoporosis, then occurring with minimal trauma. Osteomalacia is more likely in the housebound, in females and in those with old gastric surgery, malabsorption syndromes or renal failure. Osteoporosis is very common especially in the very old and in females as compared to males; rheumatoid arthritis is often associated with very extreme osteoporosis, the more so if steroid therapy has been used. Pathological rib fractures are also commonly found as a result of multiple myeloma or of metastasis from cancer of lung, breast and prostate particularly, though other primary sites may occasionally be responsible. Carcinoma of the thyroid, though likely to preferentially metastasise to bone, is rare.

A girdle distribution of chest pain suggests vertebral collapse due to malignancy or osteoporosis but more rarely may be due to involvement of the vertebra by Paget's disease or pyogenic or tuberculous infection. Herpes zoster may give girdle pain and may present considerable diagnostic problems until the rash appears. Gross osteoarthritis of the thoracic spine may also give girdle chest pain.

Tietze's syndrome, pain originating from inflammation of the costochondral junction, may often prove misleading and be mistaken for angina or myocardial infarction. It is far from rare in old age, particularly in those with rheumatoid arthritis. It is readily recognised by careful palpation which shows that the pain can be reproduced by pressure over the relevant costochondral joint.

Respiratory structures

Tracheitis, occurring in association with bronchitis or viral upper respiratory tract infections, may give retrosternal soreness. Pleuritic pain, worse on full inspiration and typically accompanied by an audible friction rub, may occur in association with any type of pneumonia (including the obstructive pneumonia secondary to a carcinoma of bronchus), with pulmonary embolism or with a haemothorax due to rib fracture. Pain from chest wall disease also tends to be exacerbated by deep inspiration and may be confused with pleural pain. However, the finding of localised tenderness over deposits or fractures or marked tenderness on compression of the chest in the former case and the auscultation of a friction rub in the latter allow clinical distinction to be made.

Massive pulmonary embolism may produce non-pleuritic

chest pain having much the same character as that of myocardial infarct pain. This is the type of pain occurring in the classical and typical presentation when the patient, often after calling for a bedpan, develops severe central pressing chest pain and almost immediately collapses and dies. Such incidents present little diagnostic difficulty and equally little opportunity for effective intervention.

The heart and great vessels
Anginal pain may be diagnostically obvious when it is typical in type and can be clearly related to effort. Unfortunately many old people are poor historians and many have atypical anginal attacks so that diagnosis may not be so straightforward. Quality of the pain is far more likely to be poorly described and fail to conform to the expected tight, gripping character. The same is true of the pain of myocardial infarction and here only a minority of infarcts present with any pain at all, painless infarction being the rule and not the exception! Myocardial infarction is much more likely to present non-specifically with premonitory falls, confusion, syncope or weakness or more obviously with acute left ventricular failure, paroxysmal nocturnal dyspnoea or the onset of congestive heart failure.

Sudden severe chest pain similar to that of myocardial infarction may also be caused by dissection of the aorta but this is infrequently seen. Pain from syphilitic aneurysm of the aorta is now a considerable rarity.

As in younger age groups, genuine cardiac disease may lead to anxiety and the occurrence of chest pain due to cardiac neurosis. However, one has the impression that this occurs far less frequently in elderly patients than in the young.

The pericardium may sometimes be the origin of chest pain. Painful pericarditis may follow myocardial infarction and is occasionally seen in uraemia, rheumatoid arthritis or from direct invasion by carcinoma of the bronchus. The finding of a pericardial rub makes the diagnosis obvious. Tuberculous pericarditis and constrictive pericarditis are very rarely seen, but pyogenic pericarditis is encountered occasionally.

Chest pain in gastrointestinal disease

Oesophagitis is an important cause of chest pain in the elderly. This usually occurs in association with the sliding type of hiatus hernia which is so common in the age group. Here, herniation of the upper part of the stomach through the diaphragm means that the normal pinch cock mechanism is no longer effective so that reflux of gastric contents into the lower oesophagus may occur. Gastric acid may then give a reflux oesophagitis and produce pain behind the sternum, 'heartburn' in fact. This pain may be quite difficult to distinguish from cardiac pain but if a story of postural aggravation of the pain is elicited the diagnosis is made obvious. The most common story is that symptoms occur on lying flat and may thus wake the patient from sleep or are brought on by stooping, for example bending down to pick up things from the floor or to tie shoe laces or leaning over the bath to clean it. Reflux oseophagitis is often associated with iron deficiency anaemia as a consequence of occult blood loss from the inflamed oesophagus.

The rolling or paraoesophageal type of hiatus hernia is far less frequently found but, though not giving rise to reflux, may produce central chest pain. However, this is something of a rarity.

Uncommonly, pain from duodenal or gastric ulceration may be referred to the chest rather than epigastrium. Gallbladder disease may similarly cause diagnostic confusion. Conversely pleuritic pain may sometimes be referred to the upper abdomen.

COUGH

Cough is a frequent symptom in elderly patients even though it may be conspicuous by its absence in respiratory infections. This is particularly so in frail and already ill old people and it is presumably this very failure of the cough mechanism which makes hypostatic pneumonia the final common path of so much terminal illness in old age. The 'old man's friend' is still the gentle quietus for many an old person, antibiotic therapy having little or no influence on the course of what is more a mechanical failure than a bacteriological problem. Those who erroneously suppose that geriatricians are responsible for 'keeping old people alive' are badly mistaken. The present increase in the geriatric age group in advanced countries is due almost entirely to improved survival in childhood, youth and middle life. Despite the development of antibiotics and indeed all the other major medical advances of the past half century, male life expectation beyond the age of 65 is virtually unchanged whilst that of females has shown only the most modest improvements.

Smoker's cough is as common in old age as in earlier age groups. Mild chronic bronchitis is common, especially in old men who have been smokers, but severe bronchitis and emphysema have been largely eliminated in late middle age by the high mortality. The pitfall is to ignore cough in an old man by assuming it is merely a smoker's cough. Such old men now represent the main remaining reservoir of open tuberculous disease in the indigenous community. Tuberculous disease of all kinds is more likely to be overlooked in old age (Cole *et al.* 1974). Chest X-ray should be a routine investigation in elderly people admitted to hospital. It is called for in elderly patients at home who have chronic cough. Furthermore, sputum should be examined for tubercule bacilli wherever the disease is a possibility but too often is not included as a part of the bacteriological examination. Bronchiectasis, asthma and mitral stenosis are other possible causes of chronic cough.

The recent onset of cough is most often due to chest infections: tracheitis, acute bronchitis, lobar pneumonia, bronchopneumonias or lung abscess. Lung abscess may be due to breakdown of a carcinoma of bronchus when the wall is typically thick and irregular on chest X-ray. Thin-walled cavities may be due to breakdown of a pneumonia, particularly those caused by infection with staphylococci or Friedlander's bacillus but may occasionally be due to an inhaled foreign body such as a dislodged carious fang.

Recent cough may also be due to carcinoma of the bronchus, pulmonary embolism or pulmonary oedema.

Cough is rarely a purely psychogenic symptom but overlay is none too rare. Cough may become far more obtrusive when the doctor is within hearing range of attention-seeking old patients.

Character of the sputum

The character of the sputum is of obvious diagnostic value. Genteel old ladies are often loath to produce sputum for inspection even when they have an obviously productive cough. In contrast some old men seem to take postive delight in expectoration and a male geriatric ward on a winter's morning may resound to a veritable dawn chorus of coughing and hawking!

When sputum can be inspected, the frothy sputum of pulmonary oedema or the purulent sputum of infection help diagnosis. Blood in the sputum is especially important.

Haemoptysis

The significance of haemoptysis in old age requires changed emphasis in its differential diagnosis compared to that in youth and middle age. Tuberculosis or mitral stenosis are rare causes—so too is bronchiectasis. Commonest cause of all is pneumonia which characteristically produces rusty sputum rather than frank haemoptysis or blood-streaking of sputum. Carcinoma of bronchus is an important cause, and in old age has a less striking preponderance in males. Haemoptysis may also occur in association with pulmonary embolism. However, though pulmonary embolism is common in old age, this presentation is distinctly unusual. Slight bloodstaining resulting in pink frothy sputum is common in left ventricular failure. Occasionally, however, left ventricular failure may give rise to a sizeable frank haemoptysis; diagnostic confusion may arise if this possibility is an unfamiliar one.

7
ALIMENTARY SYMPTOMS

DRY MOUTH

Dehydration is very common in ill old people and, though a dry mouth is often observed, the patient is unlikely to complain of it nor to feel thirsty. Frail old people may have rather a poor fluid intake at the best of times and may deliberately restrict their fluid intake because of urgency or precarious urinary continence. In illness confusion and apathy may decrease their ability to secure an adequate fluid intake but a failure of the thirst mechanism also seems to be implicated. Gross dehydration may thus develop rapidly during acute illness even when care from relatives is otherwise good. The experienced geriatric nurse is well aware of the need to encourage elderly patients to drink adequately and not to rely on their own appreciation of the need for fluid. Skin turgor change in dehydration is more difficult to recognise as elderly skin is normally inelastic. It is best assessed over the masseter muscle, a failure of the lifted skin fold to recoil briskly being a reasonably reliable indicator of dehydration.

Mouth breathing in ill patients or whilst sleeping may also produce a dry mouth. Patients may complain of a dry mouth as a drug side effect or it may be a manifestation of anxiety. The drugs most often responsible for the complaint of dryness of the mouth are those with an atropine-like effect or the atropine alkaloids themselves. The older anti-parkinsonian drugs such as benzhexol and orphenadrine, the tricyclic antidepressants such as imipramine and amitriptyline, the phenothiazine tranquillisers and antihistamines may all be implicated because of such effects. Not only may such drugs lead to a complaint of a dry mouth but salivary secretion may be reduced to such an extent as to lead to the development of acute parotitis (Hodkinson & Gunther 1972), a serious complication in an ill old person.

Finally, dryness of the mouth may be due to Sjögren's syndrome occurring in association with rheumatoid arthritis, the other chief manifestation of which is dryness and irritation of the conjunctivae.

SORE MOUTH

Angular stomatitis is fairly commonly encountered. Though this may indicate iron deficiency or riboflavine deficiency its usual cause is edentulousness and ill-fitting dentures. The latter are also the commonest cause of sore gums. Glossitis has often been ascribed to vitamin deficiencies but apart from the atrophic glossitis of B_{12} deficiency these would appear to be rare (Macleod 1972). Glossitis due to monilial infection (thrush) may be seen in debilitated patients or as an aftermath of the use of broad spectrum antibiotics.

DYSPEPSIA, HEARTBURN AND WIND

Peptic ulceration is common in old age, its symptomatology being similar to that in younger age groups except that epigastric pain is less often present or less severe. Gastric ulcers more nearly equal those of the duodenum in frequency compared with the far greater preponderance of the latter in younger age groups.

Hiatus hernia with reflux oesophagitis is increasingly common with advancing age and may give heartburn and flatulence with the characteristic feature of postural aggravation of symptoms which has already been detailed. Many patients may have no dyspeptic symptoms whatsoever, but some may none the less present with iron deficiency anaemia due to occult blood loss from the inflamed oesophagus.

Gallbladder disease is also very common in old age. At post mortem gallstones may be found in about a fifth of cases. Most gallstones in old age are asymptomatic but a minority of patients may get flatulent dyspepsia with the characteristic fatty intolerance. Occasionally carcinoma of the gallbladder develops and may give rise to persistent pain in the hypochondrium; gallstones coexist in the great majority of cases.

Cancer of the stomach is another important possibility and is one of the commoner cancers in old age. Anorexia and weight loss are usually striking features but dyspepsia and flatulence are common symptoms.

Dyspepsia may be a drug side effect. Aspirin, phenylbutazone and corticosteroids are notorious gastric irritants and may induce peptic ulceration as in earlier age groups. L-dopa has dyspepsia, nausea and vomiting as its most troublesome side effects.

Occasionally, dyspepsia and flatulence may be due to gastric atony in diabetes, to gastritis in pernicious anaemia, chronic alcoholism or uraemia. Anginal pain or pain from pleurisy may be referred to the epigastrium.

ACUTE ABDOMINAL PAIN

Acute abdominal pain can give rise to considerable diagnostic difficulties in the elderly where symptomatology may so often be atypical. Furthermore the mortality and morbidity of many of the surgical causes of acute abdomen are far greater. In part this may be because pain is less striking in old age so that disease may often be more advanced at the time of presentation. However, the morbidity of surgical intervention is far greater, abdominal surgery being badly tolerated and leading to a high incidence of major complications such as post-operative chest and pulmonary embolism.

Outlook for acute surgical emergencies of the abdomen is even more adverse when pain does not occur at all as when for example peritonitis or perforation of an ulcer produce no pain.

Acute abdomen may thus be due to perforation of a peptic ulcer, acute pancreatitis, acute cholecystitis, acute appendicitis, mesenteric infarction, diverticulitis, intestinal obstruction or peritonitis. Alternatively it may be due to non-gastrointestinal lesions such as pyelitis, cystitis, renal stone or splenic infarction. More misleading causes include herpes zoster of a lower thoracic distribution or root lesions due to vertebral collapse (usually malignant), referred pain from the chest such as pleurisy, myocardial infarction, diabetic ketosis and hypercalcaemia.

Mesenteric infarction

This is not rare in old age and is caused by arterial or venous occlusion of the mesenteric vessels. This typically results in acute abdominal pain and marked deterioration in the general condition of a patient who is often already ill from some other cause. Bloody diarrhoea and nausea and vomiting often occur also. Prognosis is extremely grave and those patients who do survive a major gut resection are frequently left with a severe malabsorption syndrome and never recover satisfactory health.

Intestinal obstruction in the elderly

Of many possible causes, carcinoma of the colon, strangulated hernia and faecal impaction call for special mention. Carcinoma of the colon is very common in old age, indeed cancer of the large bowel, that is colon and rectum together, is the commonest form of cancer in the over seventies. Cancer of the left side of the colon is particularly likely to present with intestinal obstruction whereas those of the right hemicolon are more likely to present with an abdominal mass or with anaemia. Though change of bowel habit has commonly preceded these presentations it is often not of the classical alternating diarrhoea and constipation type and is all too easily overlooked in an age group where regular and trouble free bowels are a rare blessing!

Strangulated inguinal hernia is usually diagnostically obvious but it is easy to overlook strangulated femoral hernia when it takes the form of an inconspicuous mass only to be found if the hernial orifices are palpated carefully and as an invariable routine when intestinal obstruction is suspected.

Faecal impaction is a very common occurrence in old age making rectal examination an essential routine in the elderly patient. It may on occasions be so gross as to give rise to intestinal obstruction, although this is unusual and more often spurious diarrhoea is the main consequence.

NAUSEA AND VOMITING

Nausea and vomiting may occur as an accompaniment of dyspepsia in peptic ulcer. They may be very much the predominant symptoms when pyloric stenosis has developed when vomiting may be copious in amount and of a projectile character. Vomiting may be a persistent and troublesome sequel of partial gastrectomy. Cancer of the stomach is another important cause of nausea and vomiting which are typically combined with marked anorexia and weight loss whilst some dyspepsia may also occur. Nausea and bilious vomiting may be associated with gallstones when fatty intolerance and localised tenderness over the gall bladder may make the diagnosis apparent. Nausea and vomiting, especially in the mornings, can result from the chronic gastritis of alcoholism.

Nausea and vomiting occurring in combination with acute abdominal pain may indicate such diagnoses as appendicitis, acute pancreatitis, acute cholecystitis, perforation or peritonitis. Mesenteric infarction has to be considered as a possibility, whilst diabetic ketosis is a potential 'medical' cause. The recent onset of congestive cardiac failure may sometimes result in severe liver distension giving abdominal discomfort accompanied by nausea or vomiting.

Intestinal obstruction is another important differential diagnosis, aetiology having already been considered above.

When nausea and vomiting occur in association with headache there are three main possibilities. *Migraine*, though less common in old age, may still be met and the unilateral nature of the headache, the occurrence of visual zigzag symptoms and the history of past attacks make the diagnosis obvious. *Acute glaucoma* presents with nausea and vomiting, headache or pain more localised to the eye and deterioration of vision with the appearance of haloes when the patient looks at lights. This very important ophthalmic emergency needs to be promptly recognised if vision is not to be seriously jeopardised. Finally vomiting may indicate *raised intracranial pressure;* important if uncommon. Vomiting is most likely to occur in the morning and is typically projectile whilst nausea is slight or absent. Bradycardia may point to the diagnosis whilst the finding of papilloedema makes it almost certain.

Vomiting in association with diarrhoea may be due to food poisoning due to staphylococcal enterotoxin or to a viral gastroenteritis. It may also occur in mesenteric infarction, where the diarrhoea is frequently bloody, and sometimes in uraemia, liver failure or diverticulitis.

When nausea and vomiting occur alone, drug causes are particularly likely. Digitalis is without a doubt the most common offender, the drug being widely used in the elderly and giving rise to toxicity with alarming frequency. L-dopa, morphine and stilboestrol are other important examples. Uraemia should also be considered here. Simple dietary indiscretion may be responsible. Psychogenic factors also need to be considered; anxious and neurotic old people with persistent vomiting at home among their concerned and oversolicitous relatives may become miraculously symptom free as soon as they are admitted to hospital! Vomiting may be a striking feature of the presentation of brain stem infarction due to thrombosis of the posterior inferior cerebellar artery. Vomiting may be a prominent feature of Wernicke's encephalopathy.

DYSPHAGIA

Difficulty in swallowing is a symptom which should always be taken seriously in old age as it is rarely psychogenic and may often indicate serious disease. Barium swallow examination is thus called for unless an obvious case can be recognised. Perhaps the commonest cause of dysphagia in old age is some form of neurological disease affecting the swallowing mechanism. Bulbar palsy from multiple cerebrovascular accidents is most often responsible but motor neurone disease and severe Parkinson's disease are also important. Malignancy represents another major cause of dysphagia. Most often a carcinoma of the oesophagus or of the fundus of the stomach is responsible but carcinoma of pharynx or larynx or involvement of the oesophagus by direct invasion from a carcinoma of the bronchus are alternative possibilities.

Dysphagia may be a major symptom in scleroderma. Other occasional causes include sideropenic dysphagia (Plummer-Vinson or Paterson-Kelly syndrome) occurring in severe iron deficiency, achalasia, pharyngeal pouch or oesophageal diverticulum.

An important cause of difficulty in swallowing which must always be considered is oesophagitis or oesophageal stricture due to reflux, most commonly occurring as a consequence of a sliding type of hiatus hernia. Dysphagia occurring against a background of dyspepsia with postural aggravation is very likely to be from this cause. It may represent merely severe inflammatory oedema of the oesophagus but peptic ulceration of the oesophagus may be present in addition. Such cases may respond well to medical management with antacids and postural advice. Some patients may develop permanent fibrosis and stricture and may then require bougienage as a regular and permanent routine.

Minor difficulties with swallowing may sometimes only be

attributable to deterioration of neuromuscular coordination in swallowing which appears to be a common and perhaps non-pathological development in extreme old age. Barium swallow may show impaired peristalsis, increased tertiary contractions and poor oesophageal emptying. Such minor changes may underly the common complaint of old people that they have great difficulty in swallowing pills and may be a factor in the occasional case when old people have dysphagia after attempting to swallow too large a piece of food which becomes stuck in the oesophagus. Rarely, confused old people may swallow a foreign body, sometimes their own false teeth, and block the oesophagus!

JAUNDICE

Jaundice in old age is most commonly obstructive. Gallstones are most often responsible. We have already noted how frequently gallstones are present in old age and, whilst most remain totally asymptomatic, stones may pass into the common duct and become impacted so as to cause jaundice. Many are passed spontaneously with spontaneous recovery but in other cases surgical relief of obstruction becomes essential. Mild jaundice may also occur during an attack of acute cholecystitis. Alternatively, obstructive jaundice may be due to malignant disease. Classically jaundice is distinguished by being painless when due to carcinomatous obstruction in contrast to its association with biliary colic when due to gallstones. In the old this distinction is far less reliable, gallstone jaundice often being painless also. Malignant disease of the stomach or the head of the pancreas are the tumours most likely to give obstructive jaundice. Carcinoma of the gallbladder or of the common bile duct or its ampulla are occasional causes. However, massive hepatic metastases from other neoplasms may give jaundice but the finding of a huge nodular liver makes the diagnosis obvious. Finally an obstructive jaundice may be of the cholestatic type due to drugs. Chlorpromazine (largactil) is the chief offender although it is perhaps less often seen as a cause of jaundice nowadays as its unsuitability for use in elderly patients has been more widely appreciated and alternative drugs have tended to be used in its place. Anabolic steroids are among a number of other drugs which may give cholestatic jaundice but account for only the very occasional case.

Jaundice due to hepatocellular disease is far less common. Acute hepatitis is rarely seen. Cirrhosis is relatively more frequent and alcoholism is the main recognisable cause, a substantial number of cases being cryptogenic. Primary biliary cirrhosis is rare but secondary biliary cirrhosis as a result of prolonged obstruction by stone is seen occasionally.

Marked jaundice from haemolysis is distinctly uncommon. However, mild jaundice is quite commonly seen in pernicious anaemia due to associated haemolysis. Pulmonary emboli occurring in patients with congestive cardiac failure may also result in jaundice from haemolysis of the extravasated blood. Severe septicaemic infection may also give rise to haemolytic jaundice. The acquired haemolytic anaemias are rarely encountered.

Investigation of jaundice in old age closely follows that in younger patients but it is less often justifiable to make use of invasive methods of investigation such as liver biopsy.

DIARRHOEA

Diarrhoea may have many causes in old age and can be of additional importance because it may precipitate faecal incontinence and because it can give rise to very serious debility and dehydration.

Dietary indiscretion is quite often the cause of diarrhoea in elderly patients. Many foodstuffs may be implicated but bananas are perhaps the most noteworthy. Purgative abuse must always be considered. Many elderly patients have an absolute obsession about their bowels and may not always freely admit their use of laxatives. Some use heroic doses of powerful purgatives and seem surprised when a devastating attack of diarrhoea and colicky abdominal pain follow! Purgation and diarrhoea may also attend the use of suppositories containing anthracene purgatives for, as well as acting locally, such substances are absorbed systemically. Drugs given for other purposes may have unintended laxative side effects, for example magnesium trisilicate given as an antacid or sorbitol given overgenerously as a sweetener to diabetic patients.

Outbreaks of acute diarrhoea are not a rare occurrence in wards or homes for old people. It is always wise to check that these might not be due to a dietary cause or to an overenthusiastic purgative round undertaken on the ward sister or matron's initiative and without the doctor's knowledge! Staphylococcal food poisoning needs to be considered and the possibility of bacillary dysentery excluded by stool cultures. Sonne dysentery is found on occasions and can often produce a fairly mild illness. Many such epidemics remain without any convincing explanation and may perhaps be due to viral agents.

Spurious diarrhoea is extremely common and rectal examination is an essential diagnostic procedure when diarrhoea occurs in an old person. Faecal impaction is most often the cause but rectal carcinoma may also present in this way.

Acute diarrhoea may also occur as a drug side effect. Broad spectrum antibiotics may be responsible, tetracyclines being particularly troublesome. Many other drugs may occasionally give diarrhoea, ferrous sulphate being a noteworthy example.

Diverticular disease of the colon

Diverticulosis of the colon is extremely common in old age and has been attributed to the poor fibre intake in Western communities. Prevalence rates approaching 50% have been reported. Though associated with chronic constipation, the majority of cases of diverticulosis are asymptomatic. However, acute inflammation of diverticula may occur and give rise to diarrhoea and left iliac fossa pain. More serious complications may also occur such as pericolic abscess, peritonitis, internal fistula formation or intestinal obstruction but are comparatively rare. Diagnosis can be made by demonstration of diverticula on barium enema but these are such a common finding that one should not automatically assume that they are responsible for the patient's symptoms.

Diarrhoea due to cancer

Diarrhoea is an important presentation of cancer of the colorectum, obstruction giving rise to spurious diarrhoea. Sometimes, apparent diarrhoea is due to copious mucus secretion by a large papillomatous cancer of the rectum. Cancer of the stomach or pancreas may sometimes have diarrhoea as a prominent symptom.

Other causes of chronic diarrhoea

Ulcerative colitis is not rare in old age and may develop for the first time. The finding of typical loss of haustration on barium enema and of granular proctitis on proctoscopy allow its recognition. Prognosis is variable but generally poor. In contrast, Crohn's disease is a rarity. Ischaemic disease of the intestine occurs occasionally. The presentation of acute infarction of the bowel with acute abdominal pain, vomiting and bloody diarrhoea has already been described. Rather more uncommonly, chronic ischaemia of the gut may be encountered and be responsible for chronic diarrhoea, barium studies showing segmental colitis or stricture formation.

Uraemia may give persistent diarrhoea. Thyrotoxicosis has diarrhoea as a classical symptom but this seems to be unusual in elderly cases. Rare causes of diarrhoea are scleroderma, carcinoid tumours and the autonomic neuropathy of diabetes.

Malabsorption syndromes

The malabsorption syndromes, though not particularly common in old age, represent a group of less dramatic chronic diarrhoeas. Malabsorption syndrome may be a sequel of partial gastrectomy. It may also occur in association with diverticulosis of the small bowel (Clark 1972) and rarely may be due to survival of coeliac disease into old age, to ischaemic colitis or to tuberculous disease.

Psychological factors

Psychological overlay may be a feature of diarrhoea and, as with the symptom of vomiting, admission to hospital sometimes seems to lead to dramatic and immediate cessation of diarrhoea. Some chronic diarrhoeas may be entirely psychogenic although it may be difficult to discount the role of previous habitual purgative abuse in such patients.

CONSTIPATION

So many old people are preoccupied by the state of their bowels that one may fairly say that constipation is not so much a symptom, more a way of life! The taking of 'opening medicine' by elderly people is extremely common and is often a ritual of very long standing. Attempts to persuade them to discontinue it are usually quite unavailing as they become convinced that purgation is an essential of life and that a failure to have the cherished daily bowel action is a dire portent indeed.

The tendency of the elderly to have prolonged intestinal transit time, generally infrequent bowel actions and to pass hard stools of small bulk, all of which phenomena come within the general embrace of the term constipation, is mainly related to their poor intake of dietary residue. It is also contributed to by generally poor fluid intake in old age and decreased activity and poorer muscle power.

It is against this background of near universal costiveness that the complaint of constipation must be viewed. It is often necessary to attempt to distinguish a true deterioration in bowel function from the bowel preoccupation of an anxious old person. Rectal examination is an essential part of the evaluation, for a genuine complaint of constipation in an old person is so often accompanied by faecal impaction. It may also reveal the occasional case of 'constipation' which represents obstruction from a carcinoma of the rectum.

Constipation is a common complaint in depression but may occur in any condition associated with anorexia because of the reduction in food intake. Old people are more inclined to complain of constipation than anorexia in such circumstances and may need to be reminded that one cannot make bricks without straw when they press for its relief.

Myxoedema is another important cause of constipation which may be extreme. Drugs may also be relevant; the opiates are all potent causes of constipation and codeine-containing analgesics and dihydrocodeine (DF118) should be remembered in this context. Regrettably one from time to time meets the situation where spurious diarrhoea due to faecal impaction has been treated inappropriately with kaolin and morphine mixture or some such constipating preparation because rectal examination has not been done. Atropine-like drugs may also favour the development of constipation and this used to be seen with the older anti-parkinsonian drugs such as benzhexol.

Occasionally, constipation may be caused by the inhibition of defecation because of the presence of painful anal lesions such as anal fissure or haemorrhoids.

ALTERNATING DIARRHOEA AND CONSTIPATION

Alternating diarrhoea and constipation is traditionally regarded as a particularly sinister symptom combination because of its association with carcinoma of the colon or rectum. In the elderly these carcinomata are rather more likely to give rise only to an increased degree of constipation than to give the expected alternation. Alternation of diarrhoea and constipation is far more often due to either diverticulitis, to the development of spurious diarrhoea in faecal impaction or to purgative abuse in a constipated subject.

None the less, alternating diarrhoea and constipation can hardly be ignored. If impaction is excluded, the next investigational step should be sigmoidoscopy for some three-quarters of all colorectal growths occur within sigmoidoscopic range. Barium enema should not be undertaken without careful consideration as the diagnostic yield is very low for a cancer of the colon unless an abdominal mass is palpable, and many enemas in old people are technically unsatisfactory because of the difficulties of adequate bowel preparation. The examination is often taxing as well as unpleasant for the elderly patient.

INCONTINENCE OF FAECES

This distressing symptom occurs in three main situations, where there is mental abnormality, with rectal abnormalities or as a result of diarrhoea. Faecal incontinence is an accompaniment of severe diarrhoea in most elderly subjects, continence being restored once the diarrhoea subsides. As diarrhoea has already been fully discussed, this will not be considered further.

Faecal incontinence in mental disturbance

Incontinence is all too common a sequel of confusion whether this is due to an acute confusional state or is chronic as in the dementias. There is a strong relationship between the likelihood of incontinence and the severity of confusion as measured by a simple mental test score. Those who are faecally incontinent as a result of confusion usually have very low scores, for example less than 3 on a 16 point test (Denham & Jefferys 1972). Furthermore, confusion virtually always gives urinary incontinence at an earlier stage. Faecal incontinence not accompanied by urinary incontinence should not be accepted as being due to confusion therefore. Other causes should be sought. Lone faecal incontinence may sometimes occur as an apparently deliberate action in some manipulative old people however. They may occasionally use this 'weapon' to avoid discharge from hospital or to retaliate against the staff of an institution or their relatives at home.

Rectal causes of incontinence

Apart from the very occasional case with loss of rectal control due to neurological disease such as paraplegia or the mental causes discussed above, faecal incontinence is usually a result of local conditions in the anus and rectum.

Faecal impaction is of great importance. This commonly results in incontinence because of spurious diarrhoea and because the anus becomes distended by the overfilling of the rectum. Unwary use of purgatives or of liquid paraffin is likely to make matters worse; the appropriate treatment of impaction is by local measures—manual removal, suppositories and enemata.

Spurious diarrhoea due to an obstructing carcinoma of rectum is another occasional cause of incontinence. Large prolapsing piles or rectal prolapse may also result in faecal soiling or frank incontinence.

Occasionally, faecal incontinence appears to be due to very poor tone of the anal sphincter. There may often be no clear reason for this although previous surgery for haemorrhoids may sometimes be blamed.

BLEEDING FROM THE GASTROINTESTINAL TRACT
Haematemesis

The possible causes of haematemesis in old age are generally similar to those in younger adults. Bleeding from gastric or duodenal ulcers remains a major cause and, because of sclerotic vessels, may be massive and carries a generally more unfavourable prognosis. Hiatus hernia may occasionally produce a frank haematemesis, particularly when reflux has lead to a peptic ulceration of the oesophagus. More often, however, bloodstained vomitus or occult blood loss result. The gastritis of chronic alcoholism or of uraemia is also more likely to give coffee grounds vomiting as opposed to frank haematemesis. Carcinoma of stomach may give haematemesis but bleeding oesophageal varices are a rarity in old age. Haematemesis may be precipitated by aspirin, phenylbutazone or steroid therapy.

Melaena

Care must be taken to distinguish the black stool due to oral iron therapy from melaena due to blood loss. Any cause of haematemesis may also give melaena concurrently. Equally, peptic ulcers, carcinoma of the stomach or drug induced bleeding may result in melaena without accompanying haematemesis. Other important causes of melaena are bleeding from cancer of the colon or from diverticulitis.

Bloody diarrhoea

The passage of blood and mucus as opposed to melaena indicates bleeding farther down the alimentary tract. Bloody diarrhoea may occur in mesenteric embolism or thrombosis. Blood and mucopus are characteristic of ulcerative colitis but may also be seen occasionally in severe dysentery. Diverticulitis may also give diarrhoea with bloodstaining. Large papillary cancers of the rectum may give copious bloodstained mucus. Bloody diarrhoea is an unusual symptom of cancer of the colon.

Rectal bleeding

The passing of fresh blood per rectum may be due to haemorrhoids, anal fissure, stercoral ulceration due to hard faecal impaction or carcinoma of the rectum or anus.

Occult blood loss

Iron deficiency anaemia should prompt testing of the stools for the presence of occult blood loss. The occult blood tests used are sensitive and small amounts of blood from bleeding gums, from swallowed bloodstreaked sputum or from a minor anal fissure may be enough to give a positive result and perhaps mislead one to search for bleeding from the gut. Occult gut bleeding may, of course, be from any of the many causes considered above. However, hiatus hernia is a particularly common cause of occult blood loss giving rise to anaemia when there are no other gastrointestinal symptoms. Cancer of the colon is an important though less common alternative, occult blood loss being a common presentation for growths in the caecum or ascending colon where obstruction is a late development. Peptic ulcers may be painless and present in this way sometimes, and diverticulosis is another possibility.

8

URINARY SYMPTOMS

POLYURIA, NOCTURIA AND FREQUENCY

Polyuria

Polyuria, passing an increased amount of urine, may be due to excessive fluid intake, to altered renal function or to the action of diuretic substances. It should be remembered that fluid intakes in old age are generally lower than in younger age groups so that polyuria may be truly present when the measured daily output of urine is no more than might be accepted as normal in a younger person.

Excessive fluid intake is unusual as a voluntary phenomenon in old people who generally have to be persuaded to drink adequately when they are ill. However, anxious patients may sometimes take excessive amounts of fluid and habitual tea drinkers or beer drinkers may have high fluid intakes.

Polyuria may sometimes be a feature of early renal failure as a consequence of the resulting isosthenuria—secretion of urine with a relatively fixed specific gravity. However, this is more likely to be noticed as nocturia. Both nephrogenic and true diabetes insipidus are very rare in old age.

Administered diuretics may be responsible for polyuria. This will clearly give rise to a diagnostic problem only when the diuretic substance has not been given as a diuretic, for example the use of diamox in glaucoma and the social use of caffeine containing beverages and of alcohol.

Polyuria may also be due to the osmotic diuretic effect of raised blood levels of solutes excreted by the kidney. Diabetes is the most important example where polyuria due to the osmotic effect of glycosuria is a classical presenting symptom. Similarly, hypercalcaemia may give rise to polyuria.

Nocturia

Nocturia may occur in any polyuria. It may also occur simply because too much fluid is taken late in the day. Alternatively it may be irritative in nature, in which case it is often associated with frequency during the day. Such irritative nocturia is a common feature of prostatic hypertrophy, of urinary infections such as cystitis or pyelonephritis and of the 'uninhibited neurogenic bladder', mild degrees of which appear to be common in old age even where there are no abnormal neurological signs (Brocklehurst & Dillane 1966).

Frequency

Urinary frequency may be due to polyuria, to anxiety or due to irritative or obstructive lesions. The latter are the more important. Frequency is a key symptom of infections of the urinary tract which may fail to produce fever or pain. Rigors and loin pain are hardly ever seen in acute pyelitis in old age. Acute confusional states are a common accompaniment however, urinary infection being one of the most important of the differential diagnoses in such disturbances.

Frequency is also a common symptom in prostatic hypertrophy, where hesitancy, poor stream and dribbling may be associated symptoms, in contrast to urinary infection where scalding or burning dysuria may be features of the frequency. Urgency may occur in either.

Uncommonly, frequency may be due to urethral stricture, bladder calculus or to the irritative effects of a urethral caruncle or a urethritis. Frequent voiding of small amounts of urine should be remembered as a feature of chronic urinary retention with overflow.

Finally, the uninhibited neurogenic bladder may be a cause of frequency. It presumably underlies the behaviour of some demented old people who seem to spend their entire waking day in going to and from the toilet but who have no evidence of other pathology to account for frequency.

DYSURIA AND URINARY RETENTION

Dysuria as a feature of urinary infection and of prostatic enlargement has already been referred to. Prostatic enlargement is more often benign, but carcinoma of the prostate is frequent also, being one of the most common malignancies in old men. However, many cases of carcinoma of prostate may present, not with urinary symptoms, but with symptoms due to bone metastasis such as backache or 'rheumatism' or sometimes with a leucoerythroblastic anaemia due to marrow infiltration. These possibilities further underline the need to make rectal examination mandatory in all elderly patients.

Uncommon causes of 'irritable' dysuria include bladder stone, urethral caruncle, urethritis and senile vaginitis.

Retention of urine

The possibility of retention with overflow must be remembered and palpation to exclude bladder distension is necessary in investigating the cause of frequency or of dribbling incontinence. Retention may often not be accompanied by pain even when acute, and instead present with restlessness or confusion. Obstructive, drug or neurological causes need to be considered.

Obstruction may be due to prostatic enlargment or, uncommonly, stricture, stone or paraphimosis. Extrinsic obstruction due to faecal impaction is frequent and must always be excluded.

The many drugs with atropine-like actions may all precipitate retention. The tricyclic antidepressants and older anti-parkinsonian drugs are the most likely offenders. Sympatheticomimetic drugs such as ephedrine may sometimes be implicated. Far more common than these side effects however is the precipitation of urinary retention by diuretic therapy in those who already have some degree of urinary obstruction from such causes as prostatic enlargement. The rapid-acting diuretics such as lasix or ethacrinic acid are particularly likely to give trouble.

Retention of neurological origin is more often due to the reflex neurogenic bladder such as may occur acutely after a stroke or in paraplegia. An atonic neurological bladder is rare but may occur with tabes dorsalis or polyneuritis.

Retention may occur in elderly women for no very obvious reason although it may be ascribed to such rather nebulous entities as the bladder neck syndrome. Such patients are often somewhat demented so that some form of failure in voluntary initiation of micturition may perhaps be responsible. The mild atropine-like side effects of the phenothiazine tranquillisers, so often used in elderly confused patients, may also have a contributory role in some cases.

HAEMATURIA

In younger patients the distinction between 'painless' and 'painful' haematuria is often diagnostically useful. This distinction is considerably blurred in old age where pain is far more likely to be absent. None the less, the association of pain with haematuria suggests the possibility of ureteric or bladder stone whilst suprapubic discomfort or dysuria suggest urinary infection as the probable cause.

Haematuria may be due to a very large number of possible causes but neoplasia of the renal tract will always need to be considered. Renal, pelvic or ureteric tumours are occasional causes but haematuria is particularly associated with bladder papilloma or carcinoma.

Infections of the renal tract are another important cause. Haematuria may be due to pyelonephritis and is particularly likely when renal papillary necrosis complicates it as may happen in more severe attacks and especially in diabetic patients. Acute cystitis may also be responsible and occasionally this may be due to drugs not infection as in the haemorrhagic cystitis which may complicate therapy with cyclophosphamide. Renal tuberculosis is occasionally encountered in old age and has haematuria, which may be microscopic rather than frank, as an important presenting symptom.

Renal embolisation is a further important differential diagnosis. Microscopic haematuria is a common and important pointer to the diagnosis of subacute bacterial endocarditis and represents the occurrence of multiple small emboli in the kidneys. Larger renal emboli may occur in thromboembolic disease associated with cardiac mural thrombosis after myocardial infarction or thrombus on large atheromatous plaques of the aorta. They are more often associated with frank haematuria.

Diseases associated with abnormal bleeding tendencies may sometimes be responsible for haematuria. Such rare causes as thrombocytopenia or Henoch-Schönlein purpura are completely overshadowed by the frequency of anticoagulant therapy as the reason for the bleeding diathesis.

Trauma is yet another possible cause for haematuria. The commonest example in the elderly is trauma from a self-retaining catheter which has been pulled out with the bag still inflated by a confused and uncooperative patient.

Bleeding from a urethral caruncle or from a benign or malignant prostatic enlargement are other occasional occurrences. Haemoglobinurias are hardly ever seen in old age. Acute nephritis is also very uncommon so that haematuria from this cause is most unlikely.

URINARY INCONTINENCE

Incontinence of urine is a very common symptom indeed in old age. It is very strongly associated with the presence of mental impairment whether this be due to an acute or chronic confusional state or to dementia (Denham & Jefferys 1972). It is important not to jump to the conclusion that urinary incontinence is due to confusion, however, as its causation is often multifactorial and effective treatment may be possible. Confusion mostly operates through the failure of voluntary control of micturition but incontinence may in part be due to the association of uninhibited neurogenic bladder with dementia whether of senile or arteriosclerotic type. Even where confusion is responsible for urinary incontinence, improvement may often be possible by establishing a regular regime of bladder emptying.

Simple restriction of mobility may be an important factor in incontinence, particularly where there is any element of frequency or urgency due to other factors such as urinary infection, prostatism or diuretic therapy. Incontinence may often recover with mobility in ill or frail old patients. Incontinence is far more likely to occur in bed than with the patient up in a chair; another of the many reasons for minimising bed rest in geriatric practice. Incontinence may often be regained with treatment of the auxiliary factors such as urinary infection already referred to above. Retention and overflow commonly results in dribbling incontinence whilst stress incontinence is common in old women with prolapse or previous pelvic floor damage from difficult childbirth. It is likely that senile vaginitis may sometimes contribute to urinary incontinence also. The important role of faecal impaction must again be emphasised, impairment of urinary continence often resulting from it.

Continence depends on alertness; oversedation, drowsiness, stupor or coma from any cause are likely to result in loss of urinary control. Night sedation should always be reviewed when incontinence occurs only during sleep or first thing in the morning. Neurological causes of incontinence also need to be considered. The uninhibited neurogenic bladder has already been referred to and the impaired control after stroke and in bulbar palsy or paraparesis are also important.

Psychological factors may be relevant. Old people who have been put out of their routine and bewildered by admission to hospital or an institution are far more likely to be incontinent until they have had time to settle in. Poor motivation in confused, depressed or demoralised patients makes incontinence more likely. Incontinence may sometimes be deliberate as has been mentioned already in connection with faecal incontinence.

9

NEUROLOGICAL SYMPTOMS

INVOLUNTARY MOVEMENTS

Tremor

Fine tremor may be seen from anxiety or thyrotoxicosis but may be a life long constitutional feature. Hepatic coma tends to give a coarser 'flapping' tremor but is rarely seen in old age. Severely ill patients with chronic respiratory disease may occasionally be found to have tremor due to carbon dioxide retention. Rarely, tremor may be a symptom of withdrawal of alcohol or barbiturates in habituated subjects.

Rhythmic tremor

Parkinsonian tremor is often seen although it is often a rather unobtrusive aspect of the clinical picture of the disease, rigidity being predominant. Parkinsonism is usually idiopathic but some long-standing post-encephalitic cases may still be seen. Drug-induced parkinsonism is quite common and may be due to reserpine or any of the phenothiazine tranquillisers; prochlorperazine and the long-acting injectable fluphenazine being particularly likely to produce this side effect.

So-called senile tremor may be confused with parkinsonian tremor. It commonly gives jaw tremor and titubation and is a totally benign condition. Tremor is characteristically somewhat more rapid than that of Parkinson's disease and there is no associated rigidity.

Chorea

Chorea, characterised by jerky, intermittent involuntary movements, is seen occasionally in the elderly. When confined mainly to the face it is likely to be due to phenothiazine or L-dopa therapy. This facial dyskinesia is typified by grimacing facial movements. More generalised choreiform movements are usually due to senile chorea, a degenerative condition of unknown aetiology which may often be accompanied by a mild dementia. It tends to be only mildly disabling and slowly progressive in contrast with the very occasional case of Huntington's chorea surviving into the geriatric age group in which disability and dementia are severe and the prognosis highly unfavourable. Rheumatic chorea, Sydenham's chorea, appears to be excessively rare in old age. Rarely marked chorea or choreoathetosis affecting one side of the body, hemiballismus, may have an abrupt onset following a vascular accident in the midbrain. More often there may be an acute onset of milder degrees of chorea which may be bilateral.

Fasciculation

Fasciculation, fine muscular twitching visible in the superficial muscles, is encountered occasionally. It may indicate motor neurone disease especially if accompanied by fasciculation of the tongue. It may alternatively be due to any progressive lower motor neurone lesion such as a polyneuritis or a carcinomatous myopathy. Electromyography can be of diagnostic help in such instances.

In some old people minor degrees of fasciculation may be very difficult to interpret however. One needs to be sure that the patient is quite warm so as to eliminate the possibility of shivering. Wasted old people may also show muscle twitching due to myotactic irritability. Minor fasciculation of the leg muscles may perhaps be acceptable as non-pathological in the old.

ATAXIA

Cerebellar ataxia is relatively rare in the elderly. Cases of multiple sclerosis may survive into old age and rarely one sees new cerebellar lesions due either to an idiopathic cerebellar degeneration or one occurring in association with a carcinoma.

Ataxia may sometimes be quite a striking feature in hemiplegia due to cerebrovascular accident and may greatly impede rehabilitation. Ataxia of cerebellar type may occur acutely due to a cerebrovascular accident involving occlusion of the posterior inferior cerebellar artery, vomiting and vertigo typically occurring in association.

Sensory ataxia may occur in peripheral neuritis or in the subacute combined degeneration of the cord associated with B_{12} deficiency; tabes dorsalis is now a very rare cause.

Minor ataxia may commonly result from oversedation, either from the excessive use of tranquillisers or as a hangover effect of night sedation. The anti-epileptic drug phenytoin may sometimes give quite severe ataxia as a side effect. Ataxia has also been described as a feature of hypothyroidism.

An apparently grossly ataxic gait may sometimes be hysterical as has already been mentioned.

PARAESTHESIAE

The occurrence of paraesthesiae most obviously suggests neurological causes with involvement of either the peripheral nerves or of the spinal long tracts. Possible diagnoses thus include peripheral neuropathies, old herpes zoster, meralgia paraesthetica, carpal tunnel syndrome, cervical spondylosis giving paraesthesiae in the arms from root irritation or in the legs from cord damage, subacute combined degeneration, tabes dorsalis and paraparesis. Among these, only peripheral neuropathy is at all common however. In addition, temporal lobe epilepsy or migraine may very occasionally be responsible for paraesthetic symptoms of a transient nature.

Vascular abnormalities are an important alternative to the neurological causes. Vasodilatation from any cause may give rise to odd sensations or paraesthesiae. These may be quite striking during the final vasodilatory phase of an attack of Raynaud's phenomenon which may occur in association with either rheumatoid arthritis or scleroderma. Vasodilator drugs may also produce similar symptoms and vasodilator side effects, for example of nicotinic acid given as a vitamin supplement, may sometimes be forgotten and lead to diagnostic difficulty. Ergotamine may similarly produce symptoms due to vasoconstriction. Paraesthesiae may also occur in peripheral vascular disease but may be due to the development of an ischaemic neuropathy in some instances.

Tetany, which may be due to hysterical overventilation or to hypocalcaemia, may also cause paraesthesiae. They may also be part of the multiple symptomatology of hypochondriacal depressed or psychoneurotic patients. Burning paraesthesiae of the feet may be an inexplicable but persistent symptom in old people, being troublesome in bed at night.

HEADACHE AND FACIAL PAIN

Headache is less common as a symptom in old age than in younger age groups. Although one sometimes meets headache as a part of the multiple symptomatology of depressed or psychoneurotic patients, the tension headache so often complained of by younger anxious patients is quite unusual in the elderly. Migraine may persist into old age but is usually less troublesome than before and may completely disappear in some former sufferers. Migraine virtually never makes its first appearance and the first attack of headache associated with vomiting occurring in an elderly person should suggest the possibility of raised intracranial pressure though even this is not commonly met. The headache is then typically worse in the mornings and vomiting projectile and of sudden occurrence without preceding nausea.

The finding of papilloedema supports the diagnosis. Primary or secondary brain tumour may be responsible.

Perhaps the commonest cause of headache in an elderly person is cervical spondylosis. Pain is mainly occipital but may radiate forwards to the vertex. The movements of the neck are usually grossly limited and rotation of the neck exacerbates the headache.

Temporal arteritis (cranial arteritis) is an important if not particularly common cause of headache. The pain may be very severe in some cases. It may have a throbbing character and is temporal or frontal. General malaise, fever or polymyalgia rheumatica may accompany the attack and the E.S.R. is usually considerably elevated. A thickened, tender and non-pulsating temporal artery is characteristic and biopsy showing a giant cell arteritis confirms the diagnosis. Prompt steroid therapy is indicated in view of the risk of sudden blindness due to occlusion of the central retinal artery.

Herpes zoster commonly affects the ophthalmic division of the fifth cranial nerve and may give rise to pain before the appearance of the rash a few days later. Diagnosis is obvious once the vesicular rash in the area of the nerve division has appeared. Considerable constitutional upset or fever may be present whilst the rash is at its height. Although most patients lose their pain over the succeeding week or two, an unfortunate minority are left with persistent pain—post-herpetic neuralgia. This may give unrelenting and severe pain and often irritation and is often very demoralising to the sufferer. Therapy is often disappointingly ineffective.

Glaucoma may present with headache, blurring of vision, halo formation and vomiting. It is discussed more fully under 'failing vision' in Chapter 10.

Other causes of headache such as bone metastases, middle ear infection, sinusitis or meningitis are rare. Subarachnoid haemorrhage is an occasional cause of severe headache associated with neck stiffness and often some impairment of consciousness. Toxic headache due to drugs may occasionally be encountered.

Facial pain

Trigeminal neuralgia (tic doloureux) is the most important cause, the disease most often being seen in late middle life or in old age. It is characterised by paroxysmal attacks of severe, lancinating pain of short duration—perhaps thirty seconds or so. Lacrimation and flushing of the face may occur during the attack but in between attacks there are no abnormalities to be seen. The pathognomonic feature of trigeminal neuralgia is the presence of 'trigger areas', stimulation of which precipitate attacks. Such slight stimulation may be needed that the patient is afraid to wash or shave that area of the face. Treatment with carbamezepine (Tegretol) tends to be very successful although drowsiness and dizziness may be troublesome side effects. Otherwise injection or resection of the trigeminal ganglion may give permanent relief with very small operative risk.

Other causes of facial pain are infrequently met. Arthritis of the temporo-mandibular joint may give facial pain on mastication and dental disease may give pain referred to the face. Acute parotitis gives pain which is worse on salivation and is obvious diagnostically because of the marked parotid swelling. It usually affects debilitated and dehydrated patients. Drugs with atropine-like actions favour its development and it is more likely to occur after broad spectrum antibiotics have been used, antibiotic resistant staphylococci being the usual infecting organisms.

INSOMNIA

Old people generally sleep for fewer hours than younger adults. If bored and inactive old people fall asleep for long periods by day they may, not unsurprisingly, find it difficult to sleep soundly throughout the night but may, however, expect to do so.

Having disposed of such misguided expectations, the elderly patient complaining of difficulty in sleeping needs to be regarded as a diagnostic challenge and not an occasion for the unthinking prescription of a hypnotic as symptomatic treatment.

It is helpful to go into the details of the sleep difficulty. Difficulty in getting off to sleep may be due to such environmental factors as lack of warmth and comfort, extraneous noise or unfamiliar surroundings. The alerting actions of too much caffeine in tea or coffee taken in the evening may be relevant. Intrinsic factors such as pain, itching, breathlessness, anxiety or confusion may be responsible. Broken sleep may be due to pain, orthopnoea, nocturia, cough, cramp or jumping legs. It may be due to the onset of increased nocturnal confusion in dementia or a confusional state. It may be due to bad dreams, perhaps occurring as a side effect of one of the diazepine sedatives.

Finally, the problem may be that of early waking and this is a classical symptom of depression.

DISORDERS OF SPEECH

Dysphasia

Dysphasia may be defined as a defect in the formulation, expression or understanding of spoken language. *Dysphasia* strictly refers to a partial and *aphasia* to a total inability but common usage has almost totally eroded this distinction and the two terms are used interchangeably. The same is true of an- and dysarthria, a- and dyspraxia and a- and dysphonia.

Dysphasia results from lesions of the speech area in the parietotemporal cortex of the dominant hemisphere. Dysphasia is thus associated with left hemisphere lesions in virtually all right handed patients. It used to be thought that right hemisphere lesions gave dysphasia in left handed patients but even here left sided lesions are responsible in perhaps half of cases. Other difficulties involving the use of symbols may be associated with dysphasia. These include difficulty in reading (dyslexia) and writing (dysgraphia), in using number (dyscalculia) and in the use of musical notation (amusia) for example. Dysphasia is classified into two main types; expressive dysphasia where the difficulty is predominantly in speaking and receptive dysphasia where understanding of speech is impaired. It is doubtful whether either may be 'pure', classification merely indicating which is predominant. When dysphasia is mainly receptive, monitoring of speech and insight are impaired and verbal diarrhoea (logorrhoea) and fluent but meaningless speech (jargon dysphasia) may result. These features sometimes lead to diagnostic error, the patient being thought mad.

The diagnosis of dysphasia more usually presents no great diagnostic difficulties however, particularly when it occurs acutely along with an obvious stroke and hemiplegia. Greater difficulties may arise when there is no accompanying hemiplegia, a cerebrovascular accident presenting purely as a sudden disorder of speech. A more difficult diagnostic problem is in distinguishing between dementia and dysphasia when both coexist for stroke may give considerable intellectual loss as well as dysphasia. Assessing dementia in the presence of dysphasia then becomes a real problem as all verbal tests are clearly invalidated and non-verbal tests may be too if there are symbolic difficulties. At the other extreme, the speech of severe dements may show minor dysphasic features such as word finding difficulty and perseveration but the distinction from genuine dysphasia is usually obvious.

It is easier to overlook dysphasia when it has a gradual onset. Sometimes cerebral thrombosis may give rise to dysphasia which is progressive over a few days, the so-called ingravescent stroke picture. This is in contrast to the more usual onset over the period of an hour or two in cerebral thrombosis, the more rapid onset in cerebral haemorrhage and the virtually instantaneous onset in cerebral embolism. When the onset of dysphasia is spread over more than a few days this strongly suggests the possibility of it being due to a cerebral tumour or cerebral metastases but subdural haematoma or cerebral abscess are sometimes responsible for such a presentation. A slow onset of this kind will usually indicate the need for fuller investigation therefore.

Transient dysphasia may sometimes be a feature of epilepsy

or migraine attacks and may also be seen during transient ischaemic attacks.

Dyspraxia

Dyspraxias are conditions where there is an inability to synthesise simple coordinated movements (which remain unaffected) into a more complex total pattern. They are usually a feature of parietal lesions but sometimes temporal lobe lesions may be responsible. They may thus occur together with dysphasia. Constructional apraxias may be readily demonstrated by tests involving simple constructional models or drawings, e.g. asking the patient to draw a flower or a house or a clock-face. Speech dyspraxia leads to poorly articulated speech even though there is no paresis of facial, tongue or bulbar muscles. Dyspraxias are an essentially motor phenomenon but are often associated with a corresponding agnosia, i.e. a loss of the ability to synthesise and interpret sensory information.

Dysarthria

Dysarthria implies impairment of the articulation of speech from any cause but is commonly restricted in usage so as to apply only to articulatory difficulties of neuromuscular aetiology.

Dysarthria is very common in the elderly, being far more often seen than dysphasia. It may occur in any condition affecting power and coordination of the muscles involved in the articulation of speech, i.e. the facial, tongue and bulbar muscles. Pyramidal or extra-pyramidal lesions are most often responsible, lower motor neurone or muscular causes being relatively uncommon. Facial weakness due to Bell's palsy is the commonest example from the latter category, peripheral neuropathy, myasthenia gravis or myopathies being rare causes in old age.

Pyramidal lesions frequently give dysarthria. Strokes often produce dysarthria in association with the resulting hemiplegia though this may often greatly improve with time. Bilateral strokes producing the picture of pseudobulbar palsy usually give considerable dysarthria. The syndrome, consisting of dysarthria, dysphagia, emotional lability and a spastic bilateral limb weakness, is easily recognised. Motor neurone disease is less common and gives a similar picture but with the addition of lower motor neurone lesions to the pyramidal involvement. Muscle wasting and fasciculation of limb or tongue muscles differentiate it from vascular pseudobulbar palsy. Transient dysarthria as a feature of transient ischaemic attacks may aid their differentiation from other types of 'queer turn'.

Parkinson's disease is another common cause of dysarthria and produces a recognisably different sounding speech, with monotonous tone and the frequent presence of some accompanying dysphonia with very poor volume. Chorea may also give minor dysarthria.

Cerebellar lesions are an uncommon cause of dysarthria in the elderly. The majority of the few cases seen represent the survivors of multiple sclerosis into old age. Cerebellar dysarthria affects particularly the rhythm of speech giving so called scanning speech.

Dysarthric speech from non-neuromuscular causes is often encountered in the old. Edentulousness and ill-fitting dentures are perhaps the most frequent cause. Sedation or alcohol may lead to slurring speech as may the very dry mouth of severe dehydration or Sjögren's syndrome.

Dysphonia

Dysphonia comprises weakness, hoarseness or other abnormal quality of voice. Minor dysphonic changes are usual in old age, very few old people having a voice which is not obviously recognisable as old. These 'normal' changes presumably result from normal ageing changes in strength of musculature, elasticity of the larynx and characteristics of resonating structures. The 'piping' voice of old age thus has a characteristically higher pitch, poorer pitch control and thinner resonance.

Gross dysphonic changes may be found in a variety of diseases. The weak, monotonous voice in Parkinson's disease has already been mentioned. Myxoedema may give a very characteristic dysphonia typified by deep croaking voice which is slow and monotonous and has a minor added dysarthric element. Hoarseness may be due to heavy smoking, chronic bronchitis or habitual vocal misuse when of long standing. Its recent development may be due to recent upper respiratory tract infection but may be an important presenting symptom of carcinoma of the larynx. Hoarseness associated with a bovine cough due to right recurrent laryngeal palsy from invasion by carcinoma of the bronchus is occasionally encountered.

Severe deafness may be accompanied by very characteristic voice changes. Volume is very loud and unvaried and the voice is raucous and nasal.

10

THE SPECIAL SENSES

DEFECTS OF VISION

Impairment of vision quite often develops in later life and may all too readily be accepted as a symptom of age. It is important that the patient's medical attendant does not take the same view. Many different pathologies may be responsible and a good proportion of situations are potentially remediable.

Gradual failure of vision

A gradual deterioration in vision is by far the most common complaint. This may be due to no more than a refractive error, perhaps remaining uncorrected because the incapacitated or housebound old person may not be able to obtain regular advice from his optician. In very incapacitated old people in institutional care the difficulty may simply be that of adequate cleaning of the spectacle lenses. Presbyopia (long sightedness due to difficulty in focusing on near objects because of increased rigidity of the lens) is the most common refractive problem in the elderly.

The development of cataract is another very common reason for gradually failing vision in an old person. This may be due to senile cataract or cataract associated with diabetes. Morphologically the two are identical but diabetes perhaps merely accelerates ageing changes in the lens which otherwise are largely related to hereditary factors. Nuclear cataract, perhaps to be regarded as a normal age change, is due to increasing hardness, opacity and refractive index of the centre of the lens due to an exaggerated accumulation of central lens fibres. It tends to progress very slowly and to affect mainly distance vision. Cortical cataract, in contrast, is due to localised degeneration of lens fibres resulting in patchy, dense opacities which often form radial wedges at the periphery of the lens. At an early stage, their peripheral situation may give little interference with vision but, as opacities become more extensive and involve the pupillary area of the lens, severe visual loss may result. Cortical cataracts tend to progress more rapidly than nuclear. Ophthalmoscopy allows the ready diagnosis of cataract. Surgical treatment has become increasingly refined and can be offered to quite frail old people with an acceptable small risk. Modern intracapsular operations do not impose the need for cataracts to 'mature' as did the old extracapsular techniques, and improved corneal suturing methods mean that bandaging of the eyes with its attendant risk of severe psychiatric upsets is unnecessary and that elderly patients can be remobilised within a day or two of operation. Powerful biconvex 'pebble' lenses need to be worn after cataract extraction and the distortion and magnification change which results may be difficult for an old person to adjust to sometimes. Cataract extraction is, none the less, of great potential value to the elderly person with failing vision due to cataract and should be seriously considered even in the frail.

Increasingly small pupillary size in old age coupled with opacification of the lens leads to a considerable reduction in the amount of light admitted to the eye. Old people may thus often find that their vision is seriously impaired when illumination is poor and yet may have quite good vision in brighter light.

Degenerative conditions of the retina may be responsible for progressive impairment of vision. Diabetic retinopathy, arteriosclerotic retinopathy and hypertensive retinopathy may all be encountered but the advanced retinopathy of malignant hypertension is very rarely seen in old age. Senile macular degeneration is quite common and unfortunately is not amenable to treatment. It is thought to be due to arteriosclerotic vascular changes in the choroid and may be recognised ophthalmoscopically by clumping of pigment sometimes accompanied by white scarring around the fovea. Senile macular degeneration may lead to a serious impairment of central vision but spares peripheral vision so that total blindness does not result.

Chronic glaucoma is another important possibility. Chronic simple glaucoma is relatively common and consists of a slow and insidiously increasing intraocular pressure leading to a progressive impairment of vision if unrelieved. It is associated with myopia and with age. The diagnosis is made on the findings of cupping of the optic disc, typically arcuate field defects and of raised intraocular tension on tonometry. Chronic simple glaucoma relates to deficient drainage of aqueous humour associated with open angle between the cornea and ciliary body and is perhaps due to some abnormality of the outflow channels. Its treatment is essentially medical with miotic agents such as pilocarpine and acetazolamide (Diamox) to reduce aqueous humour secretion.

Progressive visual loss accompanied by optic atrophy or papilloedema may be seen occasionally as a presentation of intracranial space occupying lesions such as a meningioma in the chiasmal region. Optic atrophy due to demyelinating disease hardly ever presents in old age.

Other uncommon causes of gradual impairment of vision include tobacco amblyopia which responds well to therapy with vitamin B_{12} given in the form of hydroxocobalamine.

Sudden deterioration of vision

Sudden and severe loss of vision of one eye suggests either some form of vascular occlusion or retinal detachment. Occlusion of the central artery of the retina and sudden loss of the vision of an eye have already been mentioned as an important presentation of cranial arteritis (Chapters 4 and 9). Ophthalmoscopic appearances are undramatic consisting of some retinal oedema, small vessels and the 'cherry red spot' if the macula is involved. The association of headache, fever or muscular pains and stiffness, point to the diagnosis, this must be made promptly so that steroid therapy is started at once to avoid loss of vision in the other eye.

Repeated episodes of transient visual loss, amaurosis fugax, may occur in association with disease of the internal carotid artery but this is quite rare. Venous thrombosis of retinal vessels may also occur occasionally and tends to produce striking ophthalmoscopic changes with large flame-shaped haemorrhages. Fortunately the visual loss is usually less severe than with arterial lesions.

Retinal detachment is more common in the old. Degenerative changes in the vitreous and in the retina itself appear to be responsible. Adhesions to the retina pull on it and may give the warning symptom of lightning flashes before detachment occurs. Minor trauma typically precipitates the detachment. Prompt surgical treatment may give useful restoration of vision.

Acute glaucoma is another important possibility. This form of glaucoma is associated with angle closure and calls for skilled emergency management and surgical treatment to improve drainage of the anterior chamber. Acute glaucoma is due to a rapid rise in intraocular tension which leads to severe pain in the eye or head, nausea and vomiting, conjunctival oedema leading to halo formation around lights and rapidly deteriorating vision. A dilated pupil which is unresponsive to light characterises the fully developed attack. The attack may sometimes have been precipitated by drugs with atropine-like actions or the use of mydriatics for some purpose.

Cerebrovascular accidents may also give acute visual defects. Hemianopia commonly occurs in strokes giving hemiplegia although the loss is often not appreciated by the patient but is noted during his rehabilitation when he tends to collide with obstacles on his hemiplegic side. Cortical blindness may result from bilateral occipital infarcts but is very rarely seen.

Other abnormalities of vision

Lightning flashes in incipient retinal detachment have already been mentioned. Zigzag flashing lights may be commonly complained of as a part of a migraine attack, whilst 'floaters', moving spots or patches, may be caused by vitreous opacities.

Double vision may represent true diplopia when two distinct images are seen or may be less accurately used to describe other minor perturbations of vision associated with fatigue, vertigo or unsuitable spectacles. True diplopia implies an ocular palsy. In old age these may sometimes be seen as part of the sequelae of a brainstem cerebrovascular accident but may less often be due to an intracranial space-occupying lesion. Isolated ocular palsies may be inexplicable and may represent vascular occlusion in the vasa nervorum. Such isolated cranial nerve palsies occur particularly in those with diabetes.

Ptosis may also represent a brainstem cerebrovascular accident and may be bilateral occasionally. Horner's syndrome, consisting of ptosis, a constricted pupil and enophthalmos, is occasionally seen. It may be associated with medullary lesions, damage to the first thoracic nerve root or involvement of the sympathetic chain in the neck but may occur as an isolated sign which remains unexplained.

Thyrotoxicosis or other thyroid disease may give rise to exophthalmic ophthalmoplegia but this is seen infrequently despite the considerable prevalence of thyroid disease in the age group.

Sore eyes

Many local lesions such as conjunctivitis may give sore eyes but several conditions are particularly common in the aged. Entropion and ectropion are both more common and may give chronic irritation. Involvement by herpes ophthalmicus may give severe conjunctivitis and sometimes corneal ulceration so that tarsorrhaphy may be needed to protect the eye. Gritty irritating discomfort of the eyes is commonly due to Sjögren's syndrome associated with rheumatoid arthritis and resulting in a keratoconjunctivitis sicca.

DEAFNESS

The prevalence of impaired hearing rises markedly with age, deafness being particularly common in old men. Hearing loss is most commonly the result of deterioration occurring progressively over many years and may be due to several types of pathology, more than one of which may be combined in the individual case.

Sensorineural deafness is particularly common and important. Its higher prevalence in men may perhaps reflect the greater importance of occupational noise as an aetiological factor in their case, recognised when extreme by such terms as 'boilermaker's deafness'. However, sensorineural hearing loss appears to be an almost inevitable ageing change which is exaggerated in some individuals whether by hereditary or extrinsic factors. As the name implies, sensorineural deafness is thought to be due to a combination of degenerative changes in both the cochlea and the auditory nerve. It typically results in preferential loss of high frequency hearing and unfortunately it is these higher frequencies which are particularly important in the understanding of speech, the consonants, on which understanding principally hinges, giving high-pitched sounds. Compensation for this high frequency loss by lip-reading and other use of visual clues is of great importance so that those with poor vision fare very badly. The phenomenon of recruitment may add to the disabilities of sensorineural deafness. It comprises a sudden change from very faint to painfully loud with a slight increase in sound volume at some critical level.

Conductive deafness may be due to chronic otitis media, otosclerosis or sometimes to arthritis of the ossicles in rheumatoid arthritis. Ageing changes altering the compliance of the conductive system may also be responsible for lesser degrees of conductive loss. Blocking of the external auditory meatus by wax is of great importance because it is very common and so eminently treatable; auriscopy should never be omitted as a part of the assessment of a patient who complains of deafness especially if there has been recent deterioration.

Paget's disease may give severe nerve deafness due to foraminal encroachment affecting the auditory nerve; calcitonin therapy does not usually lead to any improvement in hearing unfortunately. Myxoedema may also have deafness as a presenting symptom and this may be quite severe. Here, fortunately, there is usually a rapid improvement in hearing when thyroxine replacement therapy is instituted.

Deafness in one ear may be an important aspect of the presentation of *acoustic neuroma* which is not very common but is important to recognise promptly in view of the need for surgical treatment to prevent more serious deterioration. The other typical accompaniments of the progressive loss of hearing in one ear are facial weakness and loss of the corneal reflex on the same side and the development of homolateral cerebellar signs, nystagmus and dysarthria. There may also be contralateral pyramidal signs and the signs and symptoms of raised intracranial pressure.

Permanent deafness may sometimes follow the use of ototoxic drugs of which dihydro-streptomycin is the most important example. The use of this antibiotic and of streptomycin itself (which gives vestibular damage rather than hearing loss) should be totally avoided in old age, unless essential to the treatment of tuberculosis, the elderly being far more vulnerable to these disastrous side effects.

The possibility that a patient's complaint that there has been a recent deterioration in his hearing may be due to worsening of his vision rather than his hearing needs to be remembered. The visual loss, by adversely affecting the ability to lip-read and use visual clues, may lead to a marked deterioration in the ability to understand speech even though hearing is unchanged.

TINNITUS

Tinnitus, the hearing of subjective noises in the head or ears, is a common symptom in old age and is more common in elderly women. It often causes considerable distress because of its persistence and its ability to interfere with sleep. Uncommonly, the noise may be due to a vascular bruit and then may have a machine like pulsing character. More usually, the noise arises within the auditory system itself and may have a variety of qualities variously described as rushing, hissing, ringing and so on. Tinnitus is usually, but by no means invariably, associated with deafness. The deafness may be from any cause but the pitch of the tinnitus may correspond to the maximum audiometric loss and thus is typically high pitched in the common sensori-neural deafness. Tinnitus may sometimes occur as a drug side effect as for instance in salicylate overdosage.

Tinnitus is usually present in Menière's disease. This is rather uncommonly seen but may be severely disabling. There is considerable deafness and, unusually, this involves predominantly low frequency loss. The disease progresses by a series of exacerbations with partial remissions between them but may proceed to almost total deafness quite rapidly. The attacks also give rise to severe vertigo. The pathology of Menière's disease is characterised by a distension of the endolymphatic system of the inner ear but the aetiology is obscure. The disease has its peak incidence in middle life and only rarely starts beyond the age of seventy.

11
THE SKIN

PRURITUS

Itching is a fairly common symptom in old age. It may occur in the absence of any obvious rash or may be associated with a variety of dermatological diseases where there is obvious skin pathology. Irrespective of its causation, itching is accompanied by rubbing and scratching which, whilst they give temporary relief, may result in the perpetuation of the symptom because of the trauma to the skin. The psychological state of the patient thus has considerable relevance. Itching is less when attention is distracted in any way, consequently itching is often most troublesome at night. Severe pruritus lasting for some length of time quite often leads to the patient becoming demoralised, depressed or anxious.

Generalised pruritus without a rash

The commonest form of generalised pruritus in old age is senile pruritus. This seems to be related to the increased dryness of the skin in old age and the skin may be noticed to be rough and dry with fine adherent scaling. Pruritus is often more troublesome in winter, 'winter itch', because of the effects of additional drying and defatting of the skin by wind or the low humidity resulting from central heating. The itching is often brought on by the cooling of the skin which occurs when undressing. Simple emollient applications and avoidance of too great a use of soap and water usually give relief.

Less commonly, generalised pruritus may be associated with constitutional illness. The severe pruritus occurring in obstructive jaundice is the most striking example, but other conditions which may give rise to generalised itching are uraemia, myxoedema, polycythaemia rubra vera and the reticuloses.

The possibility of arthropod infestations needs to be remembered. Occasionally one meets cases of scabies in neglected old people and failure to make the diagnosis promptly may result in a minor epidemic of the disease in the hospital ward to which the patient has been admitted. The characteristic burrows should always be looked for and are most often found in the interdigital clefts and flexures, especially the ante-cubital flexure of the elbow. Generalised itching is more infrequently due to pediculosis.

Pruritus associated with rashes

Generalised itching may occur in many skin diseases as an incidental feature. It is often a striking feature in drug rashes and in exfoliative dermatitis. More localised itching may often result from intertrigo. This is very commonly seen in obese old women, particularly under the breasts and in the groins, and gives rise to areas of erythematous, macerated and malodorous skin.

Persisent severe itching may sometimes be a feature of postherpetic neuralgia and may be very difficult to relieve.

Pruritus ani

Pruritis ani may be a particularly disturbing form of localised pruritis and often interferes with sleep. Though sometimes apparently of psychogenic aetiology, it is more usually associated with local conditions such as anal fissure, haemorrhoids, monilial infection (usually occurring after the use of broad spectrum antibiotics) or maceration following use of liquid paraffin as a laxative.

Pruritus vulvae

Pruritus vulvae may be similarly disabling. It may occur in diabetes, sometimes as the presenting symptom. Alternatively, local conditions such as intertrigo, atrophic vaginitis, vaginal discharge and monilial infection may be responsible.

Pruritis vulvae may also be associated with the vulval epithelial changes leukoplakia, kraurosis vulvae and lichen sclerosus. In all of these there is hyperkeratosis of the vulval epithelium and all are premalignant conditions, squamous carcinoma of the vulva developing in perhaps 5% of cases.

PURPURA

Purpura consists of bleeding in the skin and thus includes small punctate lesions referred to as petechiae as well as extensive extravasations termed ecchymoses. Purpuric lesions do not blanch on pressure and so are readily distinguished from vascular lesions such as telangectases.

Senile purpura

Senile purpura is commonly found in the higher age groups and is most typically seen as large ecchymoses on the dorsum of the hands and backs of the forearms. It may also be seen on the sides of the face and neck. All these are areas exposed to sunlight and solar irradiation is probably an important factor in the collagen atrophy which underlies the pathology of the condition. This atrophy leads to loss of support of small vessels in the skin so that these easily rupture when subjected to shearing force and the resulting bleeding can then spread relatively widely. The ecchymosis is then readily visible through the thin atrophic skin.

Senile purpura is thus an entirely benign phenomenon which is more likely to be seen in the very old, particularly when they have any associated disease such as rheumatoid arthritis which favours skin atrophy or have been on steroid therapy.

Purpura, usually in the form of fine petechiae, may sometimes indicate thrombocytopenia. This may be due to a primary idiopathic purpura or may be secondary to leukaemia or aplastic anaemia. Thrombocytopenia may also result in other abnormal bleeding such as haematuria. Bleeding diatheses involving the clotting mechanisms do not usually give purpura.

Scurvy occurs occasionally in elderly patients, typically in less domesticated old men living alone who may subsist on bizarre diets providing virtually no vitamin C. Extensive ecchymoses in the thighs are an important feature of the presentation. Perifollicular haemorrhages and broken corkscrew hairs may also be seen. Bleeding from the gums is rarely seen as it does not occur in the edentulous who comprise the majority in older age groups.

Septicaemic conditions are another important possibility. Subacute bacterial endocarditis may give petechial rashes as well as haematuria and should always be considered when a cardiac murmur is heard. Petechial rashes may also occur in uraemia and can represent a toxic effect of drugs. Polyarteritis nodosa and Henoch-Schönlein allergic vasculitis are very rarely the cause of purpura in old age.

BLISTERS

Blisters may arise from a variety of causes. Perhaps the commonest cause of all, and certainly one which causes considerable diagnostic confusion, is the occurrence of large blisters on oedematous legs. This is quite a common occurrence in old people with considerable leg oedema from any cause. Most often this is due to cardiac failure and blistering seems particularly likely to occur when, because of orthopnoea, the patient sleeps sitting in a chair so that hydrostatic pressure in the legs remains unrelieved throughout the twenty-four hours. Typically one or more bullae develop on the front of the shins or dorsum of the foot. These are thin, tense and filled with oedema fluid, they rupture easily and leave an oval superficial ulceration. They may reach a considerable size, some being several inches in diameter, but less commonly many small blebs may form instead. These oedema blisters are rarely mentioned in textbooks or in the literature. They appear to be simply the result of prolonged elevation of hydrostatic pressure acting on the aged skin. However, though very familiar to geriatricians, they appear to be little recognised by other doctors who commonly suppose that they result from a burn from sitting too close to the fire even though their location often makes this explanation most implausible.

Small blisters are seen sometimes in the hemiplegic limb. These seem to be related to trauma, perhaps from lying on the paralysed limb, but disuse oedema of the limb may also be a factor.

Bullous lesions may occur in a number of generalised skin conditions such as dermatitis herpetiformis and erythema multiforme but two skin diseases are of particular relevance in old age, pemphigus and pemphigoid, both having blisters as their most typical lesions and both being relatively common in the elderly.

Pemphigus vulgaris

Pemphigus has its maximum incidence in middle life but is not rare in old age. It is a serious disease which had a very high mortality before steroid therapy became available and even now has a mortality of perhaps 40%. It is characterised by bullae arising on apparently normal skin, the splitting being intraepidermal so that the lesions can be pushed along the skin. Furthermore, apparently normal epidermis can be made to slide on the deeper layers of the skin by the application of sliding pressure (Nikolsky's sign). The disease appears to have an autoimmune basis, antibodies to components of stratified epithelium being demonstrable. Bullae may initially only form in the mouth but after a month or longer are found more widely, the scalp, face, pressure areas, nail folds, axillae and groins being favoured sites. The bullae readily ulcerate leaving crusted erosions. Considerable constitutional upset and weight loss are associated with the illness.

Pemphigoid

Pemphigoid is very much a disease of old age where it is about twice as frequent as pemphigus. It is a more benign disease which tends to be self-limiting and can be well controlled by steroid therapy. In contrast to pemphigus, the bullae are subepidermal not intraepidermal so that Nikolsky's sign is not present. The bullae are tense and large and either absorb to leave an erythematous patch or ulcerate and heal rapidly. Oral lesions may occur but are seldom the earliest manifestation. Typically the bullae first appear on the limbs and may remain localised for some months. Generalisation then tends to occur within a week or so. Constitutional upset, if present, tends to be slight.

12

SYMPTOMS DUE TO DRUGS

Adverse reactions to drugs are an important cause of symptoms in any age group but are of even greater importance in the elderly where the incidence of such effects is far higher (Hurwitz & Wade 1969). Adverse effects are also far more likely when the number of different drugs being taken is larger. This is of considerable relevance to the elderly where the tendency to have multiple diseases all too readily leads to the prescription of multiple treatments. The hazards of multiple prescribing are increased by the likelihood that confused or forgetful old patients will make errors in taking the drugs.

The adverse effects of drugs may arise in many different ways and any classification is somewhat arbitrary and will be used here merely as a framework for further discussion.

Overdosage

Adverse effects may arise from too large a dose of the drug. Such overdoses are more likely to occur in old age than in younger adults and there are three main reasons. Firstly, the patient is far more likely to make errors in taking his drugs because of confusion, forgetfulness or poor vision leading to misreading of instructions or misidentification of tablets. Such errors are far more likely when multiple drugs are prescribed and when regimes are more complicated—yet complex prescribing is frequently the lot of the elderly patient.

Secondly, even when the drug is taken as prescribed there may be a problem of overdose because higher blood and tissue levels are achieved by the 'normal' dose than in a younger patient because of the lower lean body weight, slower metabolism of the drug or impaired renal excretion in the older patient. Thirdly, renal function shows a gentle fall off with age but in addition to such 'normal' decline of renal function, many old people have renal disease or pre-renal factors leading to impaired function when they are ill. Adverse effects may then occur very readily in the case of drugs mainly excreted by the kidney. As an example, very very high blood levels of streptomycin may result from conventional dosage and lead to ototoxicity. Digitalis is also largely eliminated by renal excretion and a long-tolerated maintenance dose may become toxic if renal function deteriorates because of worsening heart failure or dehydration.

Side effects

Side effects are the other known pharmacological effects of a drug which are additional to the effects for which the drug has been given. These will clearly be more of a problem if there is any degree of overdosage. Furthermore, the elderly are often more vulnerable to side effects. For example, many drugs such as antihistamines, phenothiazines and tricyclic antidepressants have atropine-like side effects. These side effects are far more likely to give rise to major problems in an elderly person. Mental confusion is far more common, presumably because the elderly brain is more vulnerable because of degenerative changes. Quite serious complications such as parotitis, acute glaucoma and acute retention of urine are all more frequent, reflecting the high incidence of associated disease. The special vulnerability of the elderly mind is particularly noteworthy.

Hypersensitivity and idiosyncrasy

Hypersensitivity is when a patient has developed allergic sensitivity to a drug which has previously been administered and then developes a rash, drug fever or anaphylactic reaction on reexposure. Drug rashes are very common in the elderly to the extent that some drugs, for example ampicillin, are perhaps best avoided in elderly patients because such reactions so frequently occur. Drug idiosyncrasies are less well understood unusual reactions to a drug and may occur on first exposure to it. They include such effects as aplastic anaemia from chloramphenicol and chlorpromazine jaundice and perhaps relate to constitutional factors.

Drug interactions

Multiple drugs may interact in a variety of ways. Such interactions may lead to adverse effects and are of special relevance in old age where prescribing is so often multiple. The simplest example is perhaps that of additive effects of drugs with related actions given for different purposes, for example oversedation from the combined effects of alcohol and a night sedative. Contrary effects must also be remembered, for example the antagonism of digitalis effect by potassium supplements. More complex interactions are those due to competitive binding effects or to stimulation or inhibition of drug metabolising enzymes. These are of considerable importance in old age and call for further comment.

Competitive binding effects

Many drugs are substantially bound by serum proteins, especially by albumin. Acidic drugs binding to albumin seem to utilise the same binding sites and these have a limited capacity. There is thus competition for binding sites when two such drugs are given together and the giving of the second drug will tend to displace the first drug which is already bound and so lead to a sudden rise in its free concentration on which its pharmacological effects depend. An important example is anticoagulant therapy where the bound anticoagulant drug may be displaced by the subsequent administration of other acidic binders such as aspirin or phenylbutazone and dangerous over-anticoagulation result.

Albumin is often substantially lowered in severely ill old people so that free levels of drugs will be relatively higher and adverse effects more likely. As an example of this, Lewis and his colleagues (Lewis et al. 1971) have shown that the side effects of steroid therapy are far more frequent in patients with low serum albumin.

Enzyme induction

When some drugs which are metabolised by the liver are given for some length of time, an increased activity of the relevant microsomal enzyme systems involved in their metabolism may result. This increased enzyme activity speeds up the rate of destruction of the drug itself but also that of any other drug metabolised by the same pathway. Furthermore, the induction effect may persist for some time after the drug has been stopped. The effect of enzyme induction is thus to render the subsequent drug less effective and thus is seldom dangerous therapeutically. However, in old age enzyme induction due to the prolonged use or barbiturates as night sedatives or anti-epileptics leads to more rapid conversion of vitamin D to metabolites which are relatively inactive. As vitamin D intakes are often poor in the elderly and exposure to sunlight may be reduced or may be nil in the housebound, enzyme induction may lead to the development of osteomalacia.

Enzyme inhibition

Other drugs may inhibit certain enzyme systems. The monoamine oxidase inhibitors, such as phenelzine, nialamide and tranylcypromine, are prime examples. These antidepressant drugs owe their action to their ability to suppress the monoamine oxidase enzymes in the brain and thus increase the levels of catecholamines at the synapses and so influence mood. However, they also inhibit monoamine oxidase enzymes in other sites, those in liver being important in the detoxication of many amine compounds. Some drugs may thus have a greatly enhanced effect, for example pethidine and morphine. The impaired detoxication of other biologically active amines, such as ephedrine or amphetamines given as drugs or amines in foods such as ripe cheeses, may lead to serious toxic effects. Most dramatic of these is the precipitation of cerebral haemorrhage by their pressor effects which is particularly associated with tranylcypromine. Such hazards have discouraged the use of the monoamine oxidase inhibitor drugs in the elderly.

Indirect effects of drugs

Advese effects may arise as secondary consequences of the properties of a drug. For example, steroid therapy may reactivate chronic tuberculosis because of its anti-inflammatory effect. Many such effects consist of the precipitation of a latent disease and, as such conditions are often more prevalent in the elderly, these mechanisms are of special importance. Thus unmasking of diabetes by steroids or thiazide diuretics, precipitation of acute gout by thiazide diuretics or the induction of hypothyroidism or transient hyperthyroidism by iodides are all more likely to be seen in old age.

DRUGS ESPECIALLY ASSOCIATED WITH ADVERSE EFFECTS IN THE ELDERLY

Many adverse effects of drugs have already been referred to under the relevant symptom headings. However, those drugs and groups of drugs which are particularly troublesome in the elderly are considered further here.

Digitalis

Although of undeniable usefulness, digitalis is very much a double edged weapon, its use in old age very frequently leading to troublesome and sometimes serious adverse effects. The toxic effects are favoured by the impaired renal function and the reduced lean body mass in the old patient and 'normal' adult doses are often overdoses for elderly patients. Despite its dangers, digitalis therapy is often given to old people for inadequate reasons, particularly as maintenance therapy. Indeed Dall (1970) has shown that almost three-quarters of elderly patients could stop digitalis therapy without detriment. Concurrent diuretic therapy may enhance digitalis toxicity if hypokalaemia results because of inadequate potassium supplementation.

The toxic effects of digitalis are well known and appear to be common to all digitalis preparations. Arrhythmias are the most common, extrasystoles and coupling being particularly frequent but almost any conduction or rhythm disturbance being a possible effect. The next most common toxic effect is of anorexia and nausea. Anorexia may occur alone when the possibility of its being due to digitalis is more easily overlooked. Digitalis may also cause mental confusion. However, mental confusion is seldom seen as the first or only symptom of digitalis intoxication in my experience. Rarer manifestations include gynaecomastia and yellow vision (xanthopsia).

Diuretics

Diuretics are very widely prescribed in old age though again often for flimsy reasons. Because they are so widely used, adverse effects are seen fairly often although, provided that potassium supplementation is adequate, they are not a particularly troublesome group of drugs. The main side effect of the diuretics commonly used is potassium depletion which may lead to the insidious development of general malaise and apathy. Some diuretics are potassium sparing, for example amiloride, but here dangerous hyperkalaemia may develop in patients with poor renal function. Diuretics may be a factor in urinary incontinence or the development of urinary retention. The short acting diuretics such as frusemide are particularly likely to give rise to such troubles and a change to a slower acting drug such as chlorthalidone may be enough to obviate them. Occasionally the thiazide diuretics may precipitate acute gout or unmask latent diabetes but these effects are infrequently encountered despite the widespread use of these drugs.

Far more commonly, one may encounter dehydration or the development of hyponatraemia as results of overenthusiastic use of diuretics.

Anti-hypertensive drugs

Anti-hypertensive drugs are very likely to give rise to adverse effects in elderly patients. As there is little evidence that treatment is of benefit in mild or moderate hypertension in old age, most geriatricians tend only to prescribe these potent drugs for the rare cases of severe or malignant hypertension seen in the old. Unfortunately many other hospital doctors and general practitioners are less cautious and many old people are put in serious jeopardy by the dubiously justifiable prescription of anti-hypertensive therapy.

Two main adverse effects need to be considered, depression and hypotension. Depression is a particularly common side effect of reserpine and the depression may be severe enough to lead to suicide. There seems to be little or no justification for the use of this drug in the elderly. Its anti-hypertensive effects are too mild to make it a suitable drug for use in the more severe hypertension where treatment can be justified. Methyl dopa may similarly produce depression.

Hypotension may be a most disabling symptom and arises most readily in elderly patients. Postural hypotension may give rise to such giddiness that the patient becomes bedfast or suffers from many falls if he remains ambulant. Occasionally one sees a cerebrovascular accident occurring shortly after treatment has been initiated, presumably because of transient hypotension leading to infarction due to failure of perfusion.

Sedatives and tranquillisers

These are used on a very large scale in elderly patients. Night sedatives are often prescribed rather indiscriminately without any careful consideration of the possible reasons for insomnia. The prescription of potent night sedatives to elderly patients with unrecognised depressive illness is particularly hazardous in view of the increased suicide risk in old age. Habituation is a considerable problem; few elderly patients will readily be weaned off night sedation once this has been given for any length of time.

All night sedatives may potentiate mental confusion though the barbiturates are particularly mistrusted by geriatricians. Hangover effects are also very common so that the patient may be drowsy, apathetic and ataxic the following morning and far more likely to feel dizzy or to fall. Enzyme induction may lead to osteomalacia when barbiturate night sedation is long-term. Vivid and frightening nightmares may sometimes occur as adverse effects of nitrazepam and related drugs. Severe rashes are sometimes seen from dichloral-phenazone (Welldorm).

The tranquillisers may also potentiate confusion and may give drowsiness if dosage is too heavy. Many old people are particularly sensitive to the oversedating effects of diazepam, chlordiazepoxide and related drugs so that phenothiazine tranquilliers are generally to be preferred. The phenothiazines have many important side effects however. Cholestatic jaundice may occur with chlorpromazine. Chlorpromazine is also more likely to produce hypotension than other members of the group and for these two reasons is not a drug of first choice in old age. Anticholinergic effects are common to all members of the group and dryness of the mouth is a common symptom. Extrapyramidal side effects are particularly important. Parkinsonism may result from the use of any member of the group but is particularly troublesome with the longer acting drugs such as trifluoperazine (Stelazine), prochlorperazine (Stemetil), perphenazine (Fentazin) and the injectable fluphenazine (Modecate). Facial dyskinesia may also follow the use of phenothiazines.

An uncommon but important side effect is the facilitation of the development of hypothermia which is due to the ability of phenothiazine tranquillisers to supress shivering.

Antidepressants

The special dangers of the monoamine oxidase inhibitor drugs have already been referred to (p. 124) and are such that the tricyclic antidepressants are more often used in the elderly. These useful and widely prescribed drugs quite often give adverse effects however. They have somewhat more powerful atropine-like effects than do the phenothiazines so that dryness of the mouth and blurring of vision are quite common symptoms and rather rarely they may precipitate glaucoma or urinary retention. They quite commonly potentiate the development of postural hypotension which may give rise to giddiness or falls. Most troublesome of all are their mental side effects. Some, for example amitriptyline, may give drowsiness but all may lead to mental confusion. The full picture of acute delirium may result and agitation and hyperactivity may be specially marked. Tricyclic drugs have also been implicated in cardiac arrhythmias and in sudden unexpected death in patients with heart disease. The tricyclic antidepressants do not have extrapyramidal side effects, indeed they generally have mild anti-parkinsonian activity.

Anti-parkinsonian drugs

Parkinsonism is a common condition in old age so that these

drugs are quite often prescribed and all are rather likely to give adverse effects.

The older atropine-like anti-parkinsonian drugs have dryness of the mouth, blurring of vision and the possibility of precipitating glaucoma or urinary retention as inevitable potential side effects in view of their anticholinergic activity. Furthermore, like other cholinergic drugs, they share the ability to give rise to mental confusion. This indeed is their most frequent important side effect. Benzhexol (Artane) is particularly potent in this respect.

Amantadine (Symmetrel) has no anticholinergic activity and is a far less toxic drug. However, it occasionally results in delirious states characterised by striking visual hallucinations.

L-dopa, now the drug of choice in the treatment of Parkinson's disease, has gastrointestinal symptoms as the most common adverse effect. Nausea and vomiting are a frequent symptom and severely limit the maximum dose that can be tolerated by old people which is seldom more than 2 to 3 g per day. This restriction perhaps limits the development of other described side effects such as mental confusion, restlessness and hypersexual behaviour. Facial dyskinesia is sometimes seen however. The more recent development of combined L-dopa and carbidopa (Sinemet) makes the achievement of effective therapeutic result far easier in old patients as the gastrointestinal symptoms are generally reduced. More effective therapeutic levels can be achieved but at the price of a higher risk of the extrapyramidal side effects of L-dopa.

Antibiotics

Broad spectrum antibiotics may lead to monilial infections particularly in debilitated patients. Drug rashes occur particularly with ampicillin. Diarrhoea is quite common after broad spectrum antibiotics such as the tetracyclines because of altered bowel flora but pseudomembranous colitis may result, especially from the use of clindamycin or lincomycin. This severe form of diarrhoea has a high mortality in elderly patients (Roddis 1978). It is now known to be due to a necrotising exotoxin produced by an overgrowth of *Clostridium difficile*.

Nephrotoxicity is augmented by pre-existing renal impairment leading to high antibiotic blood levels and is important with kanamycin and the tetracyclines.

Ototoxicity with streptomycin and related antibiotics has already been mentioned (p. 112). Peripheral neuropathy sometimes occurs with the use of nitrofurantoin for prolonged periods.

Corticosteroids

The many serious potential adverse effects of steroid therapy are common to all age groups and include gastric bleeding or ulceration, impaired healing, increased susceptibility to infections and the dangers resulting from adrenal suppression. All these may be seen in old age but some effects are relatively more important. Osteoporosis is of special importance as the steroid osteoporosis will add to osteoporosis so commonly found in old age already. Gross skeletal rarefaction may thus result and lead to major disability because of spontaneous rib or vertebral fractures or femoral fracture from minor trauma. The diabetogenic effect of steroid therapy is also more likely to be seen because of the greater prevalence of latent diabetes in old people. Fluid retention may also give rise to more problems than in the young and may be enough to precipitate heart failure when added to pre-existing minor pathology.

Laxatives and purgatives

Medicine for the bowels is often demanded by elderly patients and is also a major area for self-medication. The powerful purgatives such as senna or cascara are often taken in overgenerous doses and may lead to abdominal pain and to diarrhoea with resulting dehydration and potassium depletion. Phenolphthalein is a potent sensitiser which rather often gives rashes. Liquid paraffin quite commonly leaks from the anus and gives rise to soiling and may give rise to pruritus ani because of skin maceration. More rarely it may be inhaled and give rise to a chemical pneumonia or paraffinoma and may also impede the absorption of fat-soluble vitamins. It is best avoided in old age.

SUMMARY OF SYMPTOMS DUE TO DRUGS

Anorexia	digitalis, L-dopa
Arrythmias	digitalis, isoprenaline, ANTICHOLINERGIC DRUGS: atropine, tricyclic antidepressants
Blood dyscrasias	chloramphenicol, phenylbutazone
Bronchospasm	propanolol
Cardiac failure	propanolol, fluid-retaining drugs, q.v.
Confusion	digitalis, anti-parkinsonian drugs, tricyclic antidepressants, night sedatives, tranquillisers, anti-epileptics, ephedrine
Constipation	morphia, heroin, codeine derivatives (e.g. DF118) and codeine mixtures (e.g. tab. codeine co.)
Depression	reserpine, methyl dopa, guanethidine
Diabetes	corticosteroids, thiazide diuretics
Diarrhoea	broad spectrum antibiotics, magnesium trisilicate
Drowsiness	sedatives and tranquillisers, lomotil, opiates, antihistamines, anti-epileptics
Facial dyskinesia	phenothiazines, L-dopa
Fluid retention	phenylbutazone, corticosteroids, stilboestrol, carbenoxolone
Gastrointestinal bleeding	aspirin, phenylbutazone, indomethacin, corticosteroids

Gout	thiazide diuretics
Gynaecomastia	stilboestrol, digitalis
Hypokalaemia	diuretics, carbenoxolone
Hyponatraemia	diuretics, chlorpropamide
Hypotension	phenothiazine tranquillisers, diazepam, chlordiazepoxide, tricyclic antidepressants, anti-hypertensive drugs, drugs causing hyponatraemia
Hypothermia	phenothiazines
Jaundice	chlorpromazine, anabolic steroids
Macrocytic anaemia	anti-epileptic drugs
Nausea and vomiting	digitalis, L-dopa, morphia, stilboestrol
Parkinsonism	phenothiazines, reserpine
Rashes	many drugs produce rashes occasionally, ampicillin commonly does
Respiratory depression	opiates, sedatives, CO_2 narcosis from inappropriate use of oxygen
Thyroid disorders	iodides, radiological contrast media
Vaginal bleeding	oestrogen withdrawal

REFERENCES

BAHEMUKA M, DENHAM M J & HODKINSON H M (1973) Macrocytosis. *Mod. Geriat.* **3,** 421

BAHEMUKA M & HODKINSON H M (1975) Screening for hypothyroidism in elderly inpatients. *Brit. Med. J.* **2,** 601

BANNISTER R, GILFORD E & KOCEN R (1967) Isotope encephalography in the diagnosis of dementia due to communicating hydrocephalus. *Lancet* **2,** 1014

BARRACLOUGH B M (1971) In *Recent Developments in Psychogeriatrics*, Eds. Kay D W K & Walk A, p. 87, Headley Bros.

BRITISH MEDICAL JOURNAL (1975) Epilepsy in the elderly. *Brit. Med. J.* **2,** 524

BROCKLEHURST J C & DILLANE J B (1966) Studies of the female bladder in old age, I cystometrograms in non-incontinent women. *Geront. clin.* **8,** 285

CANTOR A M (1963) A study of pernicious anaemia in elderly patients. *Geront. clin.* **5,** 23

CLARK A N G (1972) Deficiency states in duodenal diverticular disease. *Age & Ageing* **1,** 14

CLARK A N G, MANKIKAR G D & GRAY I (1975) Diogenes syndrome: a clinical study of gross neglect in old age. *Lancet* **1,** 366

COLE R B, BALMER J P & Wilson T S (1974) Surveillance of elderly hospital patients for pulmonary tuberculosis. *Brit. Med. J.* **1,** 104

COLLINS K J, DORE C, EXTON-SMITH A N, FOX R H, MACDONALD I C & WOODWARD P M (1977) Accidental hypothermia and impaired temperature homoeostasis in the elderly. *Brit. Med. J.* **1,** 353

COOPER A F, CURRY A R, KAY D W K, GARSIDE R F & ROTH M (1974) Hearing loss in paranoid and affective psychosis in the elderly. *Lancet* **2,** 851

DALL J L C (1970) Maintenance digoxin in elderly patients. *Brit. Med. J.* **2,** 705

DENHAM M J (1971) The value of blood glucose determinations as a screening method for detecting diabetes mellitus in the elderly inpatient. *Age & Ageing* **1,** 55

DENHAM M J & GOODWIN G S (1977) The value of blood cultures in geriatric practice. *Age & Ageing* **6,** 85

DENHAM M J, FARRAN H & JAMES G (1973) The value of I^{125} fibrinogen in the diagnosis of deep vein thrombosis in hemiplegia. *Age & Ageing* **2,** 207

DENHAM M J & JEFFERYS P M (1972) Routine mental testing in the elderly. *Mod. Geriat.* **2,** 275

EXTON-SMITH A N (1978) Disturbances of autonomic regulation. In *Recent Advances in Geriatric Medicine,* Ed. Isaacs B, p. 85, Churchill Livingstone, Edinburgh

FINE W (1967) Post-hemiplegic epilepsy in the elderly. *Brit. Med. J.* **1,** 199

FITZGERALD-FINCH O P & GIBSON I I J M (1975) Subluxation of the shoulder in hemiplegia. *Age & Ageing* **4,** 16

GRERO P S & HODKINSON H M (1977) Hypercalcaemia in elderly hospital inpatients: value of discriminant analysis in differential diagnosis. *Age & Ageing* **6,** 14

HODKINSON H M (1962) A study of falls and getting up from the floor in the aged. *Practitioner* **189,** 207

HODKINSON H M (1972) More favourable prognosis of motor neurone disease in old age. *Age & Ageing* **1,** 182

HODKINSON H M (1972) Evaluation of a mental test score for the assessment of mental impairment in the elderly. *Age & Ageing* **1,** 233

HODKINSON H M (1973) Mental impairment in the elderly. *J. Roy. Coll. Phycns. Lond.* **7,** 305

HODKINSON H M (1977) *Biochemical Diagnosis of the Elderly,* Chapman Hall, London

HODKINSON H M & GUNTHER H N C (1972) Drug factors in acute suppurative salivary gland infection. *Age & Ageing* **1,** 38

HODKINSON H M & POMERANCE A (1977) The clinical significance of senile cardiac amyloidosis: a prospective clinico-pathological study. *Quarterly J. Med.* **46,** 381

HODKINSON H M, STANTON B R, ROUND P & MORGAN C (1973) Sunlight, vitamin D and osteomalacia in the elderly. *Lancet* **1,** 910

HURWITZ N & WADE O L (1969) Intensive hospital monitoring of adverse reactions to drugs. *Brit. Med. J.* **1,** 531

IMPALLOMENI M G (1977) Unusual presentation of myxoedema coma in the elderly. *Age & Ageing* **6,** 71

JEFFERYS P M, FARRAN H E A, HOFFENBERG, R, FRASER P M & HODKINSON H M (1972) Thyroid function tests in the elderly. *Lancet* **1,** 924

JUDGE T G & MACLEOD C C (1968) Dietary potassium lack in the elderly. p. 295, *Proc. 5th European Meeting of Clinical Gerontology, Brussels*

KRAL V A (1962) Senescent forgetfulness: benign and malignant. *Canad. Med. Assn. J.* **86,** 257

LANCET (1970) Apathetic thyrotoxicosis. *Lancet* **2,** 809

LEWIS G P, JUSKO W J, BURKE C W & GRAVES L (1971) Prednisone side-effects and serum-protein levels. *Lancet* **2,** 778

LIVESLEY B & ATKINSON L (1974) Repeated falls in the elderly. *Mod. Geriat.* **4,** 458

MACLEOD R D (1972) Abnormal tongue appearances and vitamin status in the elderly—a double blind trial. *Age & Ageing* **1,** 99

MCMILLAN D & SHAW P (1966) Senile breakdown in standards of personal and environmental cleanliness. *Brit. Med. J.* **2,** 1032

OVERSTALL P W (1978) Falls in the elderly – epidemiology, aetiology and management. In *Recent Advances in Geriatric Medicine,* Ed. Isaacs B, p. 61, Churchill Livingstone, Edinburgh

PATHY M S (1977) Defaecation syndrome. *Age & Ageing* **7,** 233

POMERANCE A (1966) The pathology of senile cardiac amyloidosis. *J. Path. Bact.* **91,** 357

POMERANCE A (1972) Cardiac pathology in the elderly. *Mod. Geriat.* **2,** 140

PRAKASH C & STERN G (1973) Neurological signs in the elderly. *Age & Ageing* **2,** 24

RODDIS M J (1978) Antibiotic associated colitis: a retrospective study of 15 cases. *Age & Ageing* **7,** 182

SHELDON J H (1960) On the natural history of falls in old age. *Brit. Med. J.* **2,** 1685

STEVENS D L & MATTHEWS W B (1973) Cryptogenic drop attacks: an affliction of women. *Brit. Med. J.* **1,** 439
WARTENBERG R (1952) *Brit. Med. J.* **1,** 687
WILLIAMSON J, STOKOE I H, GRAY S, FISHER M, SMITH A, McGHEE A & STEPHENSON E (1964) Old people at home: their unreported needs. *Lancet* **1,** 1117

INDEX

Abdominal pain, acute 73–75
Abscess
  cerebral 55, 102
  lung 69
  subphrenic 4
Achalasia 77
Acoustic neuroma 51, 112
Addison's disease 16
Agitation 28, 30–31
Alcoholism 14, 23, 26, 33, 73, 79
  gastritis of chronic 86
  withdrawal 95
Alimentary symptoms 71–87
Anaemia 8, 18, 50, 52, 60, 62, 74, 87
  aplastic 117, 122
  iron deficiency 68, 73, 77, 87
  leuco-erythroblastic 90
  macrocytic 132
  pernicious 14, 25, 55, 73, 79
Anal fissure 83, 87, 115
Anginal pain 67
Angor animi 31
Ankylosing spondylitis 12, 38, 40, 63
Anorexia 7, 13–14, 28, 73, 125, 131
  and constipation 83

Antibiotics 129
Antidepressants 128
Antidiuretic hormone 11
Anxiety 30–31, 95
  states 14
Aorta
  aneurysm 40
  dissection 31, 67
  syphilitic aneurysm 67
Aortic
  incompetence 60
  sclerosis 60
  stenosis 53, 60
Apathy 28–30
Aphasia 101
Apnoea 64
Appendicitis, acute 74
Appetite loss 14
Arrhythmias 125, 128, 131
Arterio-sclerotic retinopathy 107
Arteritis
  cranial 108
  temporal 99
Arthritis
  hips 49
  mutilans of the hands 37
  septic 42

Arthritis (*cont.*)
   temporo-mandibular joint 100
Arthropod infestation 115
Asthma 69
   bronchial 62
Ataxia 48, 49
   cerebellar 97
Athetosis 49
Atrial fibrillation 60

Back pain 38–40
Barbiturate withdrawal 95
Behaviour, abnormal 33–34
   aggressive 33
   noisy 33
Bence Jones' proteinuria 39
Bladder
   atonic neurological 91
   papilloma 92
   reflex neurogenic 91
   stone 89–91
   uninhibited neurogenic 89, 90, 91
Blisters 117–119
Blood
   count 18
   dyscrasias 131
   loss, occult 87
Bony metastases 19, 99
Bouchard's nodes 37
Bowel infarction 81
Brachalgia due to cervical spondylosis 5, 41
Bradycardia 76
Brain
   stem
      cerebrovascular accident 110
      infarction 76

Brain (*cont.*)
   tumour 26, 99
Breath shortness 60
   at rest 61
   on exertion 62
Breathlessness, psychogenic 64
Bronchiectasis 69, 70
Bronchitis
   acute 69
   chronic 62, 69, 105
   severe 4
   tracheitis with 66
Bronchopneumonia 62, 69
   patchy 65
Bronchospasm 131

Carcinoid tumours 81
Carcinoma
   anus 87
   bladder 92
   breast 7, 37, 39, 59, 66
   bronchus 9, 16, 19, 35, 38, 41, 62, 63, 66, 68, 69, 70, 77
   colon 7, 74, 83, 86, 87, 105
   colorectum 81
   common bile duct 78
   gallbladder 73, 78
   larynx 77
   lung 7, 37, 39, 66
   oesophagus 77
   pancreas 7, 15, 59, 78
   pharynx 77, 81
   prostate 7, 37, 39, 59, 66, 90
   rectum 7, 39, 80, 83, 85, 86, 87
   stomach 7, 14, 15, 39, 73, 77, 78, 81, 86
   thyroid 66
Carcinomatosis 16, 18, 25, 40

Index

Cardiac
  amyloidosis   60
  arrhythmia   125, 128, 131
  disease   67
  failure   54, 58, 61, 62, 67, 79, 131
    cause   60
Cardio-respiratory presentations   58–70
Carotid
  artery disease, internal   109
  sinus syndrome   52
Carpal tunnel syndrome   97
Cataract   106
Causalgia   41
Cerebellar lesions   104
Cerebral
  abscess   56, 102
  embolism   56
  haemorrhage   56, 124
  thrombosis   56, 102
  tumours   11, 56
Cerebrovascular
  accident   23, 25, 26, 51, 55, 56, 97, 102, 109, 127
    brainstem   110
  disease   53
Cervical spondylosis   5, 41, 49, 97, 99
  with myelopathy   35
Chest
  infection   4, 11, 60
  pain   64, 65–68
  X-ray   17, 64, 69, 70
Cheyne–Stokes respiration   64
Cholecystitis, acute   74, 78
Chorea   43, 49, 96, 104
Choreoathetosis   45, 96
Cirrhosis   19, 59, 79
Claudication, intermittent   41, 44
Clonus, spontaneous   49

Coeliac disease   15, 82
Colitis
  ischaemic   82
  pseudomembranous   129
  ulcerative   19, 38, 81, 86
Colon, diverticulosis   80
Coma   54–57
  diabetic ketotic   56
  myxoedema   57
  non-ketotic hyperosmolar   8
Confidence, loss   13
Confusion   24–28, 67, 131
  acute   24–25
  chronic   25–26
  conditions mimicking   27
Confusional states   23, 30, 33, 48, 54, 89, 94, 101
Conjunctivae, dryness and irritation   72
Conjunctivitis   110
Consciousness, disturbed   54, 56
Constipation   82–84, 131
  chronic   80
Convulsions, epileptiform   51
Cor pulmonale   60
Cord, subacute combined degeneration   35, 45
Corticosteroids   130
Cough   64, 68–70
Cranial arteritis   99
Crohn's disease   81
Cystitis   74, 89, 92

Deafness   111–113
  severe   105
Death, self-willed   30
Debility, general   10
Deformity   43
Dehydration   71, 104
Delirium, acute   23, 24

Delusions 31
Dementia 22, 33, 48, 94, 101, 102
  arteriosclerotic 7, 26–27
  multi-infarct 7, 26
  senile 7, 15, 26–27
Dental disease 100
Dentures, swallowed 78
Depression 7, 14, 28–30, 126, 131
  constipation 82
  due to drugs 10
  hypochondriacal symptoms 3
Depressive
  illness 28–29
  symptoms 29
Dermatitis
  exfoliative 115
  herpetiformis 118
Dermatomyositis 36
Diabetes 8, 9, 16, 20, 35, 56, 73, 81, 89, 106, 110, 116, 124, 126, 131
Diabetic
  ketosis 25, 62, 74
  retinopathy 107
Diarrhoea 79–82, 129, 131
  bloody 74, 86
  due to cancer 81
  and constipation 83–84
  with vomiting 76
Digitalis 125
Disc, intervertebral, prolapsed 5, 39
Diuretics 125
Diverticular disease of the colon 80
Diverticulitis 15, 74, 76, 84, 86, 87
Diverticulosis, of small bowel 82
Dizziness 50

'Drop-attacks' 53
Drowsiness 54–57, 131
Drug
  competitive binding effects 122
  hypersensitivity 121
  idiosyncrasy 121
  interactions 122
  intoxications 55
  overdose 55, 120–121
  rashes 122
  regimens, multiple 25
Drugs
  anti-hypertensive 126
  antiparkinsonian 128–129
  side effects 9, 121
    agitation and anxiety 31
    anorexia 14
    constipation 83
    diarrhoea 129
    dry mouth 71
    enzyme induction 123
    enzyme inhibition 123
    hallucinosis 31
    headache 99
    indirect effects 124
    rashes 115, 129
    toxicity 52
Dysarthria 103
Dysentery 86
  bacillary 80
  Sonne 80
Dyskinesia, facial 46, 96, 128, 129, 131
Dyspepsia 72–73, 77
Dysphagia 77–78, 104
  sideropenic 77
Dysphasia 27, 101–103
Dysphonia 104–105
Dyspnoea 61
  diagnosis 64

Dyspnoea (*cont.*)
  paroxysmal nocturnal 63, 67
  postural 63
Dyspraxia 103
Dysrhythmia 52
Dysuria 90

Ear
  disease 50
  middle, infection 99
  wax 112
Emphysema 4, 62, 63
Empyema 4, 62
Encephalitis 56
Endocarditis, subacute bacterial
    4, 9, 60, 92, 117
Epilepsy 23, 51, 56, 102
  temporal lobe 31, 97
Erythema
  multiforme 118
  nodosum 5
Expectoration 64
Extra systoles 125
Eyes, sore 110

Face, pain 100
Faecal
  impaction 74, 80, 83, 84,
    85, 87, 90, 93
  incontinence 84–85
Faints 47–57
Falls 47–57
  fear of 13
  premonitory 47, 67
Fasciculation 96
Fatigue 16
Feet, pain 44, 50
Fever 99
Flatulence 72
Fluid retention 59, 131

Food poisoning 76
  staphylococcal 80
Foreign body
  inhaled 70
  swallowed 78
Fractures 3, 12, 17, 19
  femur 3, 12, 48
  traumatic 40
Frequency, urinary 89–90

Gait
  abnormalities 43–46, 50
  creaking 46
Gallbladder disease 73
Gallstones 78
Gastrectomy, partial 82
Gastric ulcer 72
  penetrating 40
Gastritis, chronic of alcoholism
    14
Gastrointestinal
  disease, chest pain 68
  neoplasm 15
  tract, bleeding 85–87, 131
Giant cell arteritis 99
Giddiness 13, 49–51
Glaucoma 99, 128, 129
  acute 76, 109, 121
  chronic 108
Glioma 23, 51
Glomerulonephritis 5, 20
Glossitis 72
Glucose, random 20
Glycosuria 89
Goitre, retrosternal 63
Gout 42, 44, 124, 126, 132
Gums, sore 72
Gynaecomastia 125, 132

Haematemesis 85

Haematoma, subdural 23, 26, 56, 102
Haematuria 91–92
Haemoptysis 70
Haemorrhage, subarachnoid 99
Haemorrhoids 83, 85, 87, 115
Haemothorax 66
Hallucinations 31
Hamman–Rich syndrome 63
Head injury 23
Headache 76, 98–99
Heart 67–68
  disease, ischaemic 31, 60
  failure
    congestive 25
    secondary to anaemia 25
'Heartburn' 68, 72
Heberden's nodes 37
Hemianopia 109
Hemiballismus 96
Hemiparesis, transient 55
Hemiplegia 41, 44, 46, 97, 102
Henoch-Schönlein
  allergic vasculitis 117
  purpura 92
Hepatic
  coma 95
  dysfunction 14, 26
Hepatitis, infective 4
Hepatocellular disease 79
Hernia, strangulated 74
Herpes
  ophthalmicus 111
  zoster 5, 40, 66, 74, 97, 99
  neuralgia 115
Hiatus hernia 68, 72, 77, 86, 87
Horner's syndrome 110
Hydrocephalus 26
Hypercalcaemia 16, 19, 74, 89
Hyperkalaemia 126

Hyperparathyroidism 16, 19
Hyperpnoea 64
Hypertension 60
  severe 4
Hypertensive retinopathy 107
Hyperthyroidism 8, 20, 124
Hyperventilation 41
Hypocalcaemia 41, 98
Hypoglycaemia 10, 20, 25, 31, 51, 54, 55
Hypokalaemia 11, 16, 19, 132
Hyponatraemia 10, 16, 19, 52, 126, 132
Hypopnoea 64
Hypoproteinaemia 59
Hypotension 126, 127, 132
  postural 50, 51, 128
Hypothermia 25, 56, 128, 132
Hypothyroidism 8, 16, 17, 20, 23, 124
Hysterical unconsciousness 57

Immobility 59
Incontinence
  faecal 84–85
    in mental disturbance 85
    rectal causes 85
  urinary 93–94
Infections, chronic 9
Insomnia 28, 100–101
Internal fistula formation 81
Intertrigo 115, 116
Intestine, ischaemic disease 81
  obstruction 74, 76, 81
Intoxications 55
Intracerebral disease 51
Intracranial pressure, raised 76
Involuntary movements 45, 95–96
Ischaemic attacks, transient 104

Jacksonian fits 51
Jaundice 78–79, 132
  chlorpromazine 122
  cholestatic 127
  obstructive 115
Joint
  crepitus 46
  pain 42, 44
  stiffness 44

Keratoconjunctivitis sicca 111
Ketosis 8, 56
Knee, unstable arthritic 49
Kyphoscoliosis 36, 63
Kyphosis 43
  of thoraco-lumbar spine 49

Laxatives 130
Left ventricular failure 25, 31, 54, 63, 67, 70
Leg, swollen 58–61
Leucocytosis 2, 18
Leukaemia 18, 117
Limbs, pain 40
Liver
  disease 19
  distension 76
  failure 55, 76
Locomotor and rheumatic symptoms 35–46
Looser's zones 36
Lymphangitis carcinomatosa 62

Malabsorption syndromes 82
Malaise, general 99
Malignant disease 7, 10, 36, 78
  terminal 26
Mania 34

Melaena 86
Memory impairment 21–24
Menière's disease 113
Meningioma 23, 51, 108
Meningitis 99
Mental
  alertness 48
  confusion 125, 128
    as indication of infection 2
    chest infections and 4
  symptoms 21–34
  test 22
Meralgia paraesthetica 97
Mesenteric
  embolism 55, 86
  infarction 74
Metabolic disturbances 14
Migraine 76, 97, 98, 103, 110
Mitral
  incompetence 60
  stenosis 60, 63, 69, 70
Mobility, loss 10, 11, 12
Monilial infection (thrush) 72, 115, 116, 129
Motor neurone disease 11, 35, 62, 77, 96, 104
Mouth
  dry 71, 129
  sore 72
Multiple
  disease 1–2
  sclerosis 97, 104
Muscle
  stiffness 44
  weakness 44, 62
Myasthenia gravis 16, 103
Myeloma 39
  multiple 65
Myelomatosis 18, 19, 40
  multiple 39
Myocardial infarction 41, 52, 55, 59, 61, 67, 74, 92

Myocardial infarction (*cont.*)
   painless 3
Myopathy 103
Myopia 108
Myxoedema 8, 11, 18, 23, 25, 26, 29, 32, 33, 57, 105, 112, 115
   and constipation 83
   coma 57

Narcolepsy 31, 56
Nausea 73, 74, 125, 129, 132
Nephrotic syndrome 20
Neuralgia, trigeminal 100
Neuritis, peripheral 35, 45, 48, 97
Neurological
   disorders 55
   symptoms 95–105
Neuropathy
   ischaemic 95
   peripheral 9, 12, 41, 62, 97, 103, 130
Nocturia 89

Obesity 62
Oesophageal
   diverticulum 77
   stricture 77
Oesophagitis 68, 72, 77
Oesophagus, peptic ulceration 86
Orthopnoea 61, 63
Osteoarthritis 12, 37, 38, 40, 42, 44, 46
   hips, bilateral 43
   thoracic spine 66
Osteoarthropathy, hypertrophic pulmonary 38

Osteomalacia 10, 18, 19, 36, 40, 41, 44, 65, 123, 127
Osteomyelitis 40
Osteoporosis 17, 37, 65, 66, 130
   severe generalised 38
Otitis media, chronic 112
Otosclerosis 112
Over-sedation 10, 24, 50

Paget's disease 19, 37, 40, 43, 44, 66, 112
Pain 13
   response, altered 3
Palsy
   Bell's 103
   bulbar 77, 94
   pseudobulbar 11, 35, 104
Pancreatitis 40
   acute 74
   chronic 15
Papilloedema 76
Paraesthesiae 97–98
Paralysis, general of the insane (G.P.I.) 26
Paranoid
   psychoses 30
   symptoms 32
Paraparesis 12, 48, 94, 97
Paraplegia 40, 41, 44, 85, 91
Parkinsonism 8–9, 11, 25, 26, 44, 49, 50, 54, 77, 104, 105, 128, 132
Parotitis, acute 72, 106, 121
Paterson–Kelly syndrome 77
Pediculosis 115
Pemphigoid 118, 119
Pemphigus vulgaris 118
Peptic
   perforation 74
   ulceration 72, 86, 87

Index

Pericarditis
  constrictive 59, 68
  painful 67
  tuberculous 68
Pericolic abscess 81
Peritonitis 4, 74, 81
Pharyngeal pouch 77
Pleurisy 73, 74
Plummer–Vinson syndrome 77
Pneumonia 25, 62, 66, 70
  aspiration 62
  hypostatic 54, 62, 69
  lobar 62, 69
Pneumothorax, spontaneous 61
Polyarteritis nodosa 117
Polycythaemia 18
  rubra vera 115
Polymyalgia rheumatica 35, 99
Polymyositis 36
Polyneuritis 91
Polyuria 88–89
Presbyopia 106
Pressure sores 15
Prostatic
  enlargement 90, 91, 92
  hypertrophy 89
Pruritus 114–116
  ani 115, 130
  senile 114
  vulvae 116
Pseudodementia 22, 27, 28
Psoriatic arthropathy 12, 38
Ptosis 110
Pulmonary
  embolism 52, 53, 55, 60, 61, 62, 66, 67, 70, 73, 79
  fibrosis
    chronic interstitial 63
    occupational 63
  metastases 62
  oedema 65, 70

Pulmonary (*cont.*)
  tuberculous, fibrocaseous 63
Pulse rate, increased, infection indication 3
Purpura, senile 116–117
Pyarthrosis 4
Pyelitis 74, 89
Pyelonephritis 20, 89, 92
Pyogenic infection 66
Pyramidal lesions 103

Quadriparesis 12

Radiography of chest 17
Rashes 132
Raynaud's phenomenon 17, 98
Rectal
  bleeding 87
  prolapse 85
Reiter's syndrome 12, 38
Renal
  disease 20
  failure 26, 88
    chronic 18
  papillary necrosis 92
  stone 74
  tract neoplasia 91
  tumours 91
Respiratory
  depression 132
  disease 55, 95
  infections 61
  structures 66
  tract, upper, infections 66
Responses to illness, altered 2
Reticulosis 115
Retinal
  detachment 108–109
  vessels, venous thrombosis 109
Retinopathy 107

Index

Rheumatic
  and locomotor symptoms
    35–46
  chorea 96
Rheumatoid
  arthritis 12, 19, 37, 40, 42,
    44, 46, 59, 62, 65, 66,
    67, 72, 97, 111, 116
  nodules 37
Rib fractures 17, 65, 66

Scabies 115
Scleroderma 15, 17, 77, 81, 97
Sclerosis
  aortic 60
  systemic 36
Sclerotic spinal metastases 40
Scoliosis 43
Screening tests, routine 17
Scurvy 117
Sedation 48, 127–128
Senile macular degeneration
  108
'Senility' 6
Senses, special 106–113
Septicaemia 4, 54, 79
Sexual misdemeanours 34
Shoulder
  frozen 5
  subluxation 41
Shoulder-hand syndrome 41
Simmonds' disease 57
Sinusitis 99
Sjögren's syndrome 38, 72,
  104, 111
Skin 114–119
Smoking, heavy 105
  cough 69
Speech disorders 101–105
Spine, pain 65
Splenic infarction 74
Sputum character 70

Stokes–Adams attacks 51, 52
Stomatitis, angular 72
Stone
  bladder 90, 91
  renal 74
  ureteric 91
Stroke 12, 48, 51, 52, 53, 59,
  91, 94, 102, 103
  bilateral minor 11
Stupor 54–57
Subacute combined
  degeneration 97
Subarachnoid haemorrhage 99
Sydenham's chorea 96
Syncope 52–53, 67
Syphilitic aneurism of aorta 67
Systolic murmur 60

Tabes dorsalis 45, 91, 97
Tachycardia 60
  paroxysmal 53, 61
Temperature response altered
  3
Temporal arteritis 99
Tendinopathy 38
Tetany 41, 98
Thrombocytopenia 92, 117
Thromboembolic disease 92
Thrombosis
  deep venous 58
  of posterior inferior
    cerebellar artery 51, 77
Thyroid
  disease 110
  disorders 132
  tests 20
Thyrotoxicosis 10, 16, 31, 60,
  81, 95, 110
Tic douloureux 100
Tietze's syndrome 66
Tinnitus 113

Tracheitis 66, 69
Tranquillisers 127–128
Tremor 95
   rhythmic 95
Tuberculosis 9, 69, 70
   miliary 9
   renal 92
   spinal 40
Tuberculous
   disease 82
   infection 66
   pericarditis 67
Turns 47–57
   'queer' 51–54, 104

Ulcer, gastric 72
   oesophagus 86
   peptic 55, 72, 87
   perforation 74
Ulcerative colitis 19, 38, 81, 86
Unconsciousness, hysterical 57
Uraemia 8, 16, 25, 41, 55, 59, 62, 67, 73, 76, 81, 115, 117
   gastritis 86
   progressive 14
Urea and electrolytes 18
Ureteric stone 91
Urethral
   caruncle 89, 90, 92
   stricture 89
Urethritis 90
Urinalysis 20
Urinary
   frequency 89–90
   incontinence 93–94, 126
   infection 20, 25, 89

Urinary (cont.)
   retention 90, 121, 126, 128, 129
   symptoms 88–94

Vaginal
   bleeding 132
   discharge 116
Vaginitis
   atrophic 116
   senile 90, 93
Varicose veins 58
Vascular disease, peripheral 17, 98
Venous disease 58
Vertebrae, collapsed 3, 66, 74
Vertigo 51
Vision
   blurring 129
   defects 106–111
Vitamin B_{12} deficiency 26
Vitamin D and osteomalacia 36
Vomiting 73, 74, 129, 132

Waking early 7, 28
Wandering behaviour 33
Weakness, general 16, 67
Weight loss 15, 73
Wernicke's encephalopathy 23, 77
Wheeze 64

Xanthopsia 125

Yellow vision 125